Cerebral Palsy

Guest Editor

LINDA J. MICHAUD, MD, PT

PHYSICAL MEDICINE AND REHABILITATION CLINICS OF NORTH AMERICA

www.pmr.theclinics.com

Consulting Editor
GEORGE H. KRAFT, MD, MS

August 2009 • Volume 20 • Number 3

SAUNDERS an imprint of ELSEVIER, Inc.

W.B. SAUNDERS COMPANY
A Division of Elsevier Inc.

1600 John F. Kennedy Boulevard • Suite 1800 • Philadelphia, Pennsylvania 19103

http://www.theclinics.com

PHYSICAL MEDICINE AND REHABILITATION CLINICS OF NORTH AMERICA Volume 20, Number 3
August 2009 ISSN 1047-9651, ISBN-10: 1-4377-1262-2, ISBN-13: 978-1-4377-1262-9

Editor: Debora Dellapena

Reprints. For copies of 100 or more of articles in this publication, please contact the Commercial Reprints Department, Elsevier Inc., 360 Park Avenue South, New York, NY 10010-1710. Tel.: 212-633-3812; Fax: 212-462-1935; E-mail: reprints@elsevier.com.

Physical Medicine and Rehabilitation Clinics of North America (ISSN 1047-9651) is published quarterly by Elsevier Inc., 360 Park Avenue South, New York, NY 10010-1710. Months of publication are February, May, August, and November. Business and Editorial Offices: 1600 John F. Kennedy Blvd., Suite 1800, Philadelphia, PA 19103-2899. Customer Service Office: 11830 Westline Industrial Drive, St. Louis, MO 63146. Periodicals postage paid at New York, NY and additional mailing offices. Subscription price per year is $213.00 (US individuals), $339.00 (US institutions), $107.00 (US students), $259.00 (Canadian individuals), $443.00 (Canadian institutions), $155.00 (Canadian students), $319.00 (foreign individuals), $443.00 (foreign institutions), and $155.00 (foreign students). Foreign air speed delivery is included in all *Clinics* subscription prices. All prices are subject to change without notice. **POSTMASTER:** Send address changes to *Physical Medicine and Rehabilitation Clinics of North America*, Elsevier Periodicals Customer Service, 11830 Westline Industrial Drive, St. Louis, MO 63146. **Customer Service: 1-800-654-2452 (US). From outside of the United States, call 314-453-7041. Fax: 314-453-5170. E-mail: JournalsCustomerService-usa@elsevier.com (for print support); JournalsOnlineSupport-usa@elsevier.com (for online support).**

Physical Medicine and Rehabilitation Clinics of North America is indexed in *Excerpta Medica, MEDLINE/ PubMed (Index Medicus), Cinahl,* and *Cumulative Index to Nursing and Allied Health Literature.*

Printed in the United States of America.

Contributors

CONSULTING EDITOR

GEORGE H. KRAFT, MD, MS
Alvord Professor of Multiple Sclerosis Research; Professor, Rehabilitation Medicine; and Adjunct Professor, Neurology, University of Washington School of Medicine, Seattle, Washington

GUEST EDITOR

LINDA J. MICHAUD, MD, PT
Director of Pediatric Rehabilitation and Aaron W. Perlman Professor of Pediatric Physical Medicine and Rehabilitation; Associate Professor of Clinical Physical Medicine and Rehabilitation and Clinical Pediatrics, Cincinnati Children's Hospital Medical Center, University of Cincinnati College of Medicine, Cincinnati, Ohio

AUTHORS

MINDY AISEN, MD, CEO
Adjunct Professor of Neurology, Georgetown University of Medicine; CEO, Cerebral Palsy International Research Foundation, Washington, DC

KATHARINE E. ALTER, MD
Senior Clinician, Functional & Applied Biomechanics Section, National Institutes of Health, Clinical Center; Rehabilitation Medicine Department, National Institute for Child Health and Human Development, National Institutes of Health, Bethesda, Maryland

ANITA BAGLEY, PhD
Co-Director of Motion Analysis Laboratory, Shriners Hospitals for Children, Sacramento, California

PATRICK MICHAEL BLISS, MA NACC. Cert
Staff Chaplain, Mercy Medical Center, Des Moines, Iowa

KIM VAN NAARDEN BRAUN, PhD, CDC
National Center on Birth Defects and Developmental Disabilities, Atlanta, Georgia

HENRY CHAMBERS, MD
David Sutherland Director of Cerebral Palsy Research, Rady Children's Hospital, San Diego, California

DIANE L. DAMIANO, PhD, PT
Chief of Functional and Applied Biomechanics Section, Rehabilitation Medicine Department, Clinical Center, National Institutes of Health, Bethesda, Maryland

DEBORAH GAEBLER-SPIRA, MD
Attending Physician and Professor of Physical Medicine and Rehabilitation, Department of Pediatrics, Pediatric Rehabilitation Program, Rehabilitation Institute of Chicago, Chicago, Illinois

GEORGE GORTON, BS
Director of Clinical Outcomes Assessment Lab, Shriners Hospitals for Children, Springfield, Massachusetts

CYNTHIA FRISINA GRAY, MA, MBA
Cofounder of Reaching For The Stars. A Foundation of Hope for Children with Cerebral Palsy (RFTS, Inc.), Alpharetta, Georgia

CHRISTINE MURRAY HOULIHAN, MD
Assistant Professor of Pediatrics, Department of Pediatrics, University of Virginia, Charlottesville, Virginia

ELIZABETH McCARTY, OTR/L, ATP
Clinical Coordinator and Assistive Technology Practitioner, Aaron W. Perlman Center, Cincinnati Children's Hospital Medical Center, Cincinnati, Ohio

CLAIRE MORRESS, MEd, OTR/L, ATP
Clinical Faculty, Department of Occupational Therapy, College of Social Sciences, Health and Education, Xavier University; Assistive Technology Practitioner, Aaron W. Perlman Center, Cincinnati Children's Hospital Medical Center, Cincinnati, Ohio

KEVIN P. MURPHY, MD
Medical Director, Gillette Specialty Healthcare Northern Minnesota Clinics; Medical Director, Medical Center One Pediatric Rehabilitation Center, Bismarck North Dakota; Associate Professor, Department of Physical Medicine and Rehabilitation, University of Minnesota Duluth School of Medicine; Colonel, MNARNG Medical Corps, Gillette Specialty Healthcare, Duluth, Minnesota

DONNA J. OEFFINGER, PhD
Director of Research Development, Pediatric Orthopedics, Shriners Hospitals for Children, Lexington, Kentucky

AMY THORNHILL PAKULA, MD
Department of Pediatrics, The Marcus Autism Center, Emory University, Atlanta, Georgia

DAVID W. PRUITT, MD
Assistant Professor of Clinical Physical Medicine, Rehabilitation and Clinical Pediatrics, Departments of Pediatrics, Physical Medicine and Rehabilitation, Division of Pediatric Rehabilitation, Cincinnati Children's Hospital Medical Center, University of Cincinnati College of Medicine, Cincinnati, Ohio

ERIN RIEHLE
Director of Project SEARCH and Department of Disability Services, Cincinnati Children's Hospital Medical Center, Cincinnati, Ohio

SARAH P. ROGERS, MPH
Coordinator of Clinical Outcomes Program, Shriners Hospitals for Children, Lexington, Kentucky

SUSIE RUTKOWSKI, Med
Co-Director and Educational Specialist, Project SEARCH, Great Oaks Institute of Technology and Career Development, Cincinnati, Ohio

MELISSA SIEBERT, JD, MBA
Board of Directors, Reaching For The Stars. A Foundation of Hope for Children with Cerebral Palsy (RFTS, Inc), Alpharetta, Georgia

KERSTIN SOBUS, MD
Assistant Professor, Department of Clinical Pediatrics Specialty and Pediatric Physical Medicine and Rehabilitation, Indiana University School of Medicine, Clarian Health Partners (Methodist-IU-Riley), Indianapolis, Indiana

RICHARD D. STEVENSON, MD
Professor of Pediatrics, Department of Pediatrics, University of Virginia, Charlottesville, Virginia

TOBIAS TSAI, MD
Resident Physician of Physical Medicine, Rehabilitation and Pediatrics Training Program, Departments of Pediatrics, Physical Medicine and Rehabilitation, Division of Pediatric Rehabilitation, Cincinnati Children's Hospital Medical Center, University of Cincinnati College of Medicine, Cincinnati, Ohio

CHESTER M. TYLKOWSKI, MD
Chief of Staff, Pediatric Orthopedics, Shriners Hospitals for Children, Lexington, Kentucky

JILDA VARGUS-ADAMS, MD, MSc
Assistant Professor, Departments of Pediatrics and Physical Medicine & Rehabilitation, Division of Pediatric Rehabilitation, Center for Epidemiology and Biostatistics, Cincinnati Children's Hospital Medical Center, University of Cincinnati College of Medicine, Cincinnati, Ohio

MARSHALYN YEARGIN-ALLSOPP, MD, CDC
National Center on Birth Defects and Developmental Disabilities, Atlanta, Georgia

Contents

> This article reviews the historical background, classification, and etiology
> of cerebral palsy (CP), the most common motor disability of childhood.
> The various methods employed to measure the prevalence of CP in the
> population are examined. Causes of CP are numerous, and the etiology
> multi-factorial. Risk factors are categorized by the timing of their proposed
> occurrence: prenatal, perinatal, and postnatal. The leading prenatal and
> perinatal risk factors for CP are birth weight and gestational age. Other
> risk factors include neonatal encephalopathy, multiple pregnancy, infec-
> tion and inflammation, and a variety of genetic factors.

> The medical issues associated with the diagnosis of cerebral palsy (CP)
> can have significant interplay with the neuromuscular issues that most
> physiatrists manage in the clinical setting. Identification and appropriate
> management of these common comorbidities by the primary care and
> subspecialist physicians can have significant impact on the quality of life
> of the patient and family. Some of these issues are prevalent across all
> gross motor function classification system (GMFCS) levels of severity,
> whereas others more commonly complicate the care of those children
> with the more severe GMFCS levels IV and V. Performance of a complete
> review of systems to address the potentially complex medical comorbid-
> ities and subsequent application of appropriate screening tools can assist
> in achieving optimal outcomes in children with CP and their families.

> Cerebral palsy (CP) is the most prevalent physical disability in childhood
> and includes a group of disorders with varying manifestations. This article
> focuses on current and future intervention strategies for improving mobility
> and participation during the lifespan for ambulatory children with CP. The
> provision and integration of physical therapy and medical and orthopedic
> surgery management focused primarily on the lower extremities are dis-
> cussed here. Some of the newer trends are more intense and task-related

exercise strategies, greater precision in tone identification and management, and a shift towards musculoskeletal surgery that focuses more on promoting dynamic bony alignment and less on releasing or lengthening tendons. Advances in basic and clinical science and technology development are changing existing paradigms and offering renewed hope for improved functioning for children with CP who face a lifelong disability with unique challenges at each stage in life.

This article discusses the problem of osteoporosis in cerebral palsy. Osteoporosis remains a major health problem worldwide. Cerebral palsy is the most prevalent childhood condition associated with osteoporosis. Bone density is significantly decreased. Children with cerebral palsy often sustain painful fractures with minimal trauma that impair their function and quality of life. This article addresses the anatomy and structure of bone and bone metabolism, the clinical assessment of bone mass, the causes of osteoporosis and its evaluation and treatment in children with cerebral palsy.

Advances in medical and surgical care over the past 20 years have resulted in children who formerly would have died at birth or in infancy now surviving into adulthood, many with significant, permanent physical disabilities, including those due to cerebral palsy (CP). Increased awareness of these problems is needed by adult health care providers, who will be providing direct care to these individuals, and also by pediatric providers, who may be able to anticipate and prevent some of the long-term problems. This article reviews the common medical-surgical problems and their management in adults with CP. In addition the life experience of a 44 year-old with CP is described from a personal perspective.

Children with a diagnosis of cerebral palsy often have significant physical limitations that prevent exploration and full participation in the environment. Assistive technology systems can provide opportunities for children with physical limitations to interact with their world, enabling play, communication, and daily living skills. Efficient access to and control of the technology is critical for successful use; however, establishing consistent access is often difficult because of the nature of the movement patterns exhibited by children with cerebral palsy. This article describes a 3-phase model of evaluation and intervention developed and used by Assistive Technology Services at the Aaron W. Perlman Center, Cincinnati

Children's Hospital Medical Center, to establish successful access to technology systems in children with cerebral palsy.

Susie Rutkowski and Erin Riehle

The employment statistics for people with disabilities are dismal and particularly low for those with cerebral palsy. As practitioners working with young people who have moderate to severe cognitive and physical challenges, including those with cerebral palsy, the authors assert that there are best practices that make a difference. There are states and programs showing successful outcomes. Those who create partnerships among education, businesses, and rehabilitation agencies are seeing direct positive results in employment outcomes for people with disabilities, as well as cultural and perceptional changes in businesses and people who have hiring capability. This article reviews the relevant literature; conclusions are drawn and recommendations made to improve the employment outcomes for youth with cerebral palsy in their transition to adult life.

Donna J. Oeffinger, Sarah P. Rogers, Anita Bagley, George Gorton, and Chester M. Tylkowski

This article provides an overview of outcome tools commonly used to assess ambulatory children with cerebral palsy, research findings from a recent large multi-center study, and ways to integrate the research findings into clinical practice. The information presented in this article and in the referenced articles provides information on: outcome tools' discriminatory ability and responsiveness; readily available comparison data on 7 commonly used outcome tools that can be used at the point of care; prediction equations for the Parent report Pediatric Outcomes Data Collection Instrument (PODCI) by age and Gross Motor Function Classification System (GMFCS) level; and minimum clinically important difference thresholds by GMFCS level. This information can help clinicians select the best outcome tools to discriminate among severity levels and avoid ceiling effects. The scores provided allow direct comparisons between a specific patient and a matched cohort, assisting clinicians in the creation of comprehensive and individualized evaluation and management plans. Use of appropriate outcome tools to assess children with cerebral palsy can lead to best practices and reduced costs in the clinical setting.

Jilda Vargus-Adams

Describing the status of children with cerebral palsy (CP) and quantifying change in their status are 2 central challenges to research and clinical management of CP. The science of assessing and reporting status is outcome measurement, and it is rapidly developing in the arena of CP. Because of the large number of domains to measure, the variability of CP manifestations, and a limited number of "gold standard" evaluations, creating an accurate, comprehensive, responsive, and broadly applicable measurement strategy is a serious endeavor. A range of outcome measures are available to address CP issues across the spectrum of disability. The use of these measures, and others yet to be developed, provides researchers and clinicians the best means of understanding CP and the effects of treatments.

Cynthia Frisina Gray, Melissa Siebert, Mindy Aisen,
and Deborah Gaebler-Spira

Rehabilitation management of children with cerebral palsy (CP) brings together parents and doctors. The primary goal of the contact is to improve the individual child's potential and to improve the child's functional outcomes. Frequently, parents are interested in not just their own child, but the population of children with cerebral palsy. Physicians can provide information for both purposes. Successful parent–professional relationships are rewarding and powerful. Combining the passion of the parent and the expertise of the physician can enhance collaboration for advocacy efforts that improve outcomes for children with cerebral palsy. An increasingly important component in the parent–medical collaboration is the identification of networks of local and national support for families of children with cerebral palsy. Fortunately, parents and organizations focused on children with cerebral palsy are seeing the necessity for collaboration to build community awareness, implement education programs, and spearhead pediatric cerebral palsy advocacy on a nationwide basis.

THE CLINICS ARE NOW AVAILABLE ONLINE!

Access your subscription at:
www.theclinics.com

Foreword

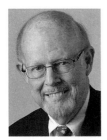

George H. Kraft, MD, MS
Consulting Editor

During its entire history, the *Physical Medicine and Rehabilitation Clinics of North America* has never had an issue dedicated to cerebral palsy (CP). I hope the reader will agree that it is time that we correct this, and that Dr Michaud is the right person to organize this important effort.

I remember that when I was in training, it seemed perplexing that we were seeing a fairly large number of children with CP, but hardly any adults. Was this because patients with CP did not survive into adulthood? Was it because the disease somehow improved over time? Or was it that CP was there all of the time, but we just did not recognize it? I know for sure that there was a stress during pediatric rehabilitation rotations on CP, whereas it was hardly seen in adult clinics.

It also seems that over the years CP is getting to be less common. This should not be surprising, as in recent years more research has become available on prevention, and more attention has been placed on pregnancy and care during childbirth.

I am pleased that these changes are reflected in this issue, and it shows why the *Clinics* continues to be so important: it serves the same purpose as a textbook, but a dynamic one. It is as if every 3 months a new and detailed chapter is incorporated into the textbook. Dr Michaud is a well-known pediatric physiatrist who has been on the faculties of the University of Washington and the University of Pennsylvania; she now heads the University of Cincinnati pediatric rehabilitation division. She has gathered together an impressive group of experts in CP to contribute to this issue, and topics included range from epidemiology to patient–professional partnerships. Starting with current CP classification, this issue of *Clinics* moves through various medical comorbidities and the latest research in lower limb management. Related topics, such as the effect of CP on bone density and the development of new technology, are covered. Function and outcomes tools are also covered. Finally—and I am very glad to see these—there are articles on caring for adults with CP and on employment issues faced by persons with CP.

Phys Med Rehabil Clin N Am 20 (2009) xiii–xiv
doi:10.1016/j.pmr.2009.06.016
1047-9651/09/$ – see front matter © 2009 Elsevier Inc. All rights reserved.

pmr.theclinics.com

I thank Dr. Michaud for accepting the guest editorship of this issue and for organizing an outstanding issue on this topic.

George H. Kraft, MD, MS
Rehabilitation Medicine
Department of Neurology
University of Washington
Box 356490
1959 NE Pacific Street, Seattle
WA 98195-6490, USA

E-mail address:
ghkraft@uw.edu (G.H. Kraft)

Preface

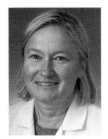

Linda J. Michaud, MD, PT
Guest Editor

Cerebral palsy (CP) is the most common condition associated with disability in childhood and is thus the number one diagnosis encountered by the pediatric physiatrist. Furthermore, as mortality is low, most children with CP will grow into adults with CP, presenting new challenges to physiatrists who will care for these individuals as adults. National and international surveillance programs have facilitated studies of prevalence and risk factors in different subgroups, and recent advances are in progress to incorporate measures of functioning into epidemiologic studies, as presented by Dr. Pakula and colleagues. At the level of the individual patient, Drs. Pruitt and Tsai take a review of systems approach to identifying and managing common medical comorbidities that frequently interact with the functional problems of children with CP. The physiatric focus on individuals with CP is often on interventions for problems in function, and Drs. Damiano, Alter, and Chambers provide an excellent update on nonoperative as well as operative interventions for the lower extremities. There is growing awareness of the problem of osteoporosis in nonambulatory children, including those with CP, and Drs. Houlihan and Stevenson review challenges in assessment of bone density and management in this population.

As pointed out by Dr. Murphy and colleagues, we have much to learn about recognizing and managing the issues facing individuals with CP across the lifespan; however, findings to date should guide early care. Access to technology and to employment and economic independence are essential considerations for the quality of life of many people with CP and their families, as presented by authors McCarty, Morress, Rutkowski and Riehle, respectively. The need for high expectations for good vocational outcomes is a recurring theme emphasized in the articles by Dr. Murphy and colleagues, and by authors Rutkowski and Riehle.

Dr. Oeffinger and colleagues present a 6-year project evaluating the performance of outcome tools in common clinical and clinical research use to assess ambulatory children with CP. They provide minimal clinically important differences for these tools stratified by levels of CP severity. This work clearly illustrates the potential to develop better evidence-based practices in the management of children with CP. Yet, as pointed out by Dr. Vargus-Adams, there remain many obstacles, related to the

Phys Med Rehabil Clin N Am 20 (2009) xv–xvi
doi:10.1016/j.pmr.2009.06.013
1047-9651/09/$ – see front matter © 2009 Elsevier Inc. All rights reserved.

pmr.theclinics.com

heterogeneity of this population across all levels of severity, that challenge our ability to evaluate the results of our interventions meaningfully. Gray and colleagues have the "last word" on parent-professional partnership, suggesting that professionals involved in the care of children with CP should move forward together with parents in furthering efforts to improve the quality of life for children with CP and their families.

Personally and professionally, I am grateful to many wonderful children with CP and their families and to many interdisciplinary colleagues, including those contributing to this issue, for shaping my experiences and inspiration over the past 35 years in my career as a physical therapist and then pediatric physiatrist.

Linda J. Michaud, MD, PT
Pediatric Rehabilitation
Cincinnati Children's Hospital Medical Center
3333 Burnet Avenue, MLC 4009
Cincinnati, OH 45229-3039, USA

E-mail address:
linda.michaud@cchmc.org (L.J. Michaud)

Cerebral Palsy: Classification and Epidemiology

Amy Thornhill Pakula, MD[a], Kim Van Naarden Braun, PhD, CDC[b],
Marshalyn Yeargin-Allsopp, MD, CDC[b],*

KEYWORDS

- Epidemiology • Cerebral palsy • Prevalence
- Risk factors • Surveillance

HISTORY AND DEFINITION

Cerebral palsy (CP) is the most common motor disability of childhood. A recent publication from the Autism and Developmental Disability Monitoring (ADDM) CP Network sponsored by the Centers for Disease Control and Prevention (CDC) reported a prevalence of 3.3 per 1000 8-year-old children from 3 sites across the United States.[1] The history of cerebral palsy is a long one, dating back to ancient Egypt. There are at least 2 drawings of individuals from the fifth century BC with what is recognized today as spastic cerebral palsy.[2,3] An orthopedic surgeon, William John Little, who himself had an equinus deformity from early childhood secondary to poliomyelitis, is credited with the first descriptions of CP in 1843.[4] Seeking a cure for his own deformity, he was greatly influenced by the French orthopedic surgeon, Jacques Delpeche, who was interested in surgical correction of equinus deformities, and performed many tenotomies of the Achilles tendon.[5] After successful correction of his own deformity by a German orthopedic surgeon, George Stromeyer, Little improved on Stromeyer's surgical techniques and set up the Orthopaedic Institution in London. Little's interest in orthopedic deformities continued and he is regarded as a pioneer in orthopedic surgery and as the first to recognize spastic paralysis. He wrote a treatise "On the influence of abnormal parturition, difficult labor, premature birth and asphyxia neonatorum on the mental and physical condition of the child", which posited that these deformities of childhood were related to anoxia secondary to trauma occurring during

The findings and conclusions in this report are those of the authors and do not necessarily represent the official position of the Centers for Disease Control and Prevention.

[a] Emory University, Department of Pediatrics, The Marcus Autism Center, 1920 Briarcliff Road, Atlanta, GA 30329, USA

[b] CDC, National Center on Birth Defects and Developmental Disabilities, MS E-86, 1600 Clifton Road, Atlanta, GA 30333, USA

* Corresponding author.

E-mail address: mxy1@cdc.gov (M. Yeargin-Allsopp).

labor and delivery.[6] For many years, spastic diplegia was commonly referred to as Little's disease.

Sir William Osler, a British physician, is believed to have coined the term "cerebral palsy" in 1889; he described 151 patients affected by the disorder.[7] Sigmund Freud, a neurologist, but best known as a psychoanalyst, wrote many articles on CP, adding to the sparse body of knowledge on the subject. He also disagreed with Little on its cause, observing that children with CP had many other neurologic conditions, such as intellectual disabilities, visual impairment, and epilepsy. He therefore believed that CP might be caused by in utero abnormalities of brain development. He divided CP into 3 groups based on possible causes: (1) maternal and idiopathic congenital; (2) perinatal; and (3) postnatal, and devised a classification scheme with "diplegia" used to refer to all bilateral disorders of central origin.[8]

The American Academy of Cerebral Palsy (AACP) was formed in 1947.[5] Minear[9] polled the membership of the Academy in 1953 and found many different definitions of cerebral palsy. The various definitions commonly acknowledged a broad syndrome of brain damage, with predominant motor dysfunction but also psychological, epileptic, and behavioral symptoms. Transient abnormalities, neoplasms, progressive disorders, and spinal cord disorders were excluded. Despite the presence of common themes, a unified definition of CP was not presented until almost 5 years later by the Little Club, an informal group of neurologists and others formed in the United Kingdom in 1957. The Little Club developed a definition aimed to facilitate sharing knowledge and research: "Cerebral palsy is a persisting qualitative motor disorder due to non-progressive interference with development of the brain occurring before the growth of the central nervous system is complete." The Little Club classification consisted of: (1) spastic (hemiplegic, double hemiplegic, and diplegic); (2) dystonic; (3) choreoathetoid; (4) mixed; (5) ataxic; and (6) atonic CP.[10] In the 1960s CP was redefined but there continued to be recognition of inconsistencies in terminology.[11]

With growing interest in public health, the Spastics Society commissioned a group to define CP for epidemiologic purposes in the 1980s. A limb-by-limb classification system, which described the functioning of each limb and the head and neck separately, built on the work in Western Australia of Fiona Stanley, was proposed by Evans.[12] This classification system also allowed the capture of information on co-occurring medical conditions such as congenital malformations and seizures. American and European CP investigators met from 1987 to 1990 and developed a common definition: "CP is an umbrella term covering a group of non-progressive, but often changing, motor impairment syndromes secondary to lesions or anomalies of the brain arising in the early stages of development."[13]

By 1998, there were 14 centers across Europe conducting population-based surveillance for CP; they formed a Network, the Surveillance of Cerebral Palsy in Europe (SCPE).[14] The Network used a case definition that was a reiteration of that of Mutch et al,[13] and developed and published standardized procedures for ascertaining and describing children with CP for registers.[14]

An International Workshop on Definition and Classification of CP was held in Bethesda, Maryland, July 11 to 13, 2004 because of a perceived need to revisit the definition and classification of CP.[15] The current definition, as adopted by this group, recognizes that CP is more than a motor disability and acknowledges that often other impairments accompany CP: "Cerebral palsy describes a group of permanent disorders of the development of movement and posture, causing activity limitation, that are attributed to non-progressive disturbances that occurred in the developing fetal or infant brain. The motor disorders of CP are often accompanied by disturbances of sensation, perception, cognition, communication, behavior, by epilepsy and by secondary musculoskeletal problems."[15]

The definitions of CP, including the most recent one cited,[15] have 4 core components: (1) it is a disorder of movement and posture; (2) it results from an abnormality in the brain; (3) it is acquired early in life; and (4) the condition is static at the time of recognition. However, there are still many challenges with the use of all CP definitions for epidemiologic purposes because of the lack of specificity of the definition. The criteria do not address severity of the motor disability to be included; how to assure that the brain abnormality is static; age of the acquisition of the brain lesion; or the youngest age of recognition of the condition.[16] Also, there are other conditions that do meet these stated criteria for CP that are not included.[17] Blair and Stanley have proposed that to make the term cerebral palsy more specific, especially for epidemiologic studies, CP researchers should: (1) define the lower limit of severity using a validated measure, such as the Gross Motor Function Classification System (GMFCS); (2) specify an upper age limit for post-neonatally acquired cases; (3) develop inclusion and exclusion criteria related to known chromosomal, genetic, and metabolic conditions; (4) define the age of certainty of the diagnosis beyond which one would not expect resolution or change in the diagnosis; and (5) define the minimum age of inclusion of the child in a register or surveillance system should the child die before diagnostic confirmation. Blair and Stanley also state that even if investigators do not agree on the same criteria for studies, a description of the study population according to the 5 areas as suggested would allow for comparison of results from different epidemiologic studies.[16]

CLASSIFICATION

In 1956 Minear and the Nomenclature and Classification Committee of the American Academy for Cerebral Palsy presented a set of potential classification schemes that have remained pertinent over the years.[9] This early classification system included broad clinical symptoms with categories for physiology (the nature of the motor abnormality), topography, etiology, neuroanatomic features, supplemental (associated) conditions, functional capacity (severity), and therapeutic requirements. Experts continue to address these broad categories when classifying CP.

Physiologic and Topographic Classification

CP can be divided into 2 main physiologic groups, the *pyramidal* (a term used somewhat inexactly to refer to cases in which *spasticity* is prominent) and the *extrapyramidal* types (chorea, athetosis, dystonia, ataxia). Spasticity is a clinical sign manifested by an increased resistance of a limb to externally imposed joint movement. The spastic types of cerebral palsy have neuromotor findings that are consistent and persistent; neurologic abnormalities remain during quiet periods and sleep, and do not vary much during the active state or when degrees of emotional stress or irritability are present. In contrast, extrapyramidal types of CP have marked variability in tone during relaxation and sleep, and especially during wakefulness when stressful situations arise. Rapid passive movement at a joint elicits spastic hypertonus. The classic descriptor of spasticity is the "clasp knife" resistance that is followed by a sudden "give." The comparison is made to the opening or closing of a penknife. Extrapyramidal hypertonicity, in contrast, is represented by increased tone persisting throughout slow passive flexion and extension of an extremity. It is often described as "lead pipe" rigidity. Combinations of these tone patterns in the same patient are common, creating potential difficulty in finding the proper diagnostic terminology. Extrapyramidal CP has 4-limb involvement, with upper extremities typically being functionally more involved than the lower extremities. This situation precludes further useful topographic breakdown. Therefore, for practical purposes topographic classification is restricted to the spastic group.

To discriminate subgroups of spastic CP, classification systems often refer to the *localization* or *topography* of the abnormal motor function. *Diplegia* refers to bilateral lower extremity involvement, *hemiplegia* to unilateral upper and lower extremity involvement, *triplegia* to involvement of 3 extremities (typically both lower and one upper extremity), *double hemiplegia* to 4-extremity involvement with more severe spasticity of the upper extremities, and *quadriplegia/tetraplegia* to severe 4-extremity involvement.

There are several concerns with the physiologic and topographic schemes. The distinction between the topographic classification terms may lack sufficient reliability.[18] How much upper extremity involvement is required to distinguish diplegia from quadriplegia? How many extrapyramidal signs are required to designate mixed CP? "Lead pipe" rigid tone is not always easily distinguished from spasticity. Alberman[19] compared agreement on classification of CP among 6 trained clinicians and found poor reliability. Agreement on the physiologic classification of the motor dysfunction (eg, spasticity, choreoathetosis) was 40%, on the topographic classification 50%, and on severity (mild, moderate, severe) 60%. In addition to reliability concerns, the topographic and physiologic classifications do not consider functional abilities. Because brain dysfunction has diffuse manifestations in childhood, each child must be evaluated thoroughly for associated impairments in areas such as learning and cognition, vision, behavior, epilepsy, and secondary neuromuscular abnormalities. It is not possible to direct clinical assessments simply based on correlations between topography and associated dysfunctions. Finally, topographic and physiologic classifications do not aid therapy.

Etiologic Classification

Etiologic classification systems are aimed at developing prevention strategies. The association of erythroblastosis fetalis with choreoathetoid cerebral palsy served as the paradigm for this classification. However, etiologic classifications are not well developed and to date have not been successful in addressing prevention.[20,21]

The Collaborative Perinatal Project[22] helped to identify a large number of conditions that placed a child at risk for cerebral palsy. However, only a few of these conditions were found to correlate to specific motor outcome or diagnosis.[23] Most predictors were combinations of factors present prior to onset of labor, implying that CP is not caused by a single disturbance but by the interaction of many related conditions.

Some research has also focused on discerning the mechanism of the brain damage.[24] Because the brain has a limited number of ways to respond to insult, CP might result from a common pathophysiological mechanism. One hypothesis links inflammatory factors and white matter damage,[25] proposing that asphyxia, maternal infection (such as urinary tract infection), and chorioamnionitis might be related to CP through a common mechanism.

Neuropathologic Classification

In the mid-twentieth century, the idea of neuropathologic classification was proposed in an effort to reflect and highlight the inability to relate brain structure to brain function. The advent of neuroimaging has not yet significantly advanced the ability to classify CP by neuropathology. Ultrasound, magnetic resonance imaging, computed tomography, and volumetric studies have not demonstrated consistent structure or functional relationships.[21] However, as science has learned more about the developing brain, a theory of selective vulnerability has developed. Two important associations have been described: (1) periventricular leukomalacia with prematurity, and (2) basal ganglia injury with term asphyxia. Newer and functional imaging techniques with different discriminatory abilities might contribute significantly to a neuropathologic classification of cerebral palsy in the future.[26]

Supplemental Classification and Associated Conditions

The supplemental classification describes the associated conditions or impairments found in children with CP and attempts to connect them to the physiologic and topographic classifications.[21] The idea is to identify syndromes that have a common etiology and ultimately lead to prevention. Bilirubin encephalopathy is a prototypical example of such a syndrome, and includes choreoathetoid cerebral palsy, vertical gaze palsy, dental enamel dysplasia, and sensorineural hearing loss. It has a predictable clinical course, with extensor spells during the first few months, followed by hypotonia, then choreoathetosis, and finally dystonia during adolescence. Despite a few such examples, the associations between supplemental disorders (associated impairments) and physiology or topography generally have low sensitivity and specificity.[21] Individuals with CP must each be evaluated for an array of associated conditions, including deficits in hearing, vision, cognition, and academic achievement.

Functional and Therapeutic Classifications

Minear and the Nomenclature and Classification Committee[9] originally added functional and therapeutic classifications for cerebral palsy simply to be comprehensive. The functional classification addresses the degree of severity of the condition based on limitation of activity. The therapeutic classification divides cases into 4 categories: nontreatment, modest interventions, need for a cerebral palsy treatment team, and pervasive support.

Much has changed with regard to therapeutic interventions since the 1950s. The number of interventions is significantly greater. Interventions are applied not only to the primary motor dysfunction but also to associated disorders or conditions. Service delivery systems have shifted from clinical or hospital settings to schools and the community. Therefore, older therapeutic classification systems have required adaptation. Capute and colleagues[27] interpreted CP as part of a broader syndrome of brain dysfunction, in turn suggesting that CP be part of a broader spectrum of motor dysfunction. They pointed out that in some cases, the most limiting factor is not the motor impairment, and that the treatment of CP should extend beyond the motor deficit to associated cognitive, communicative, convulsive, or behavioral conditions that affect therapeutic and functional (adaptive) success.

Interest in functional classifications has recently intensified due to a broader understanding of outcome. Newer measures of functional abilities in cerebral palsy have evolved. The World Health Organization International Classification of Functioning, Disability, and Health (ICF)[28] articulates three categories of function: impairment (the *capacity* to perform), activity limitations (the *ability* to perform), and participation restrictions (the *opportunity* to function).

Cerebral Palsy Classification for Epidemiologic Surveillance

Throughout the 1960s and 1970s, issues related to the classification of CP were largely addressed from a clinical perspective. However, in the 1980s, with rising interest in monitoring CP prevalence among populations as public health markers of rapidly changing neonatal care, significant consideration was given to classification of CP from an epidemiologic perspective. Evans' "limb-by-limb" classification method looked at central motor abnormalities based on neurologic type: hypotonia, hypertonia (including stiffness, spasticity, and rigidity), dyskinesia, and ataxia.[12] This classification method included information on each limb, the head and neck, functional mobility and manual dexterity, as well as associated conditions (intellectual and sensory impairments, communication problems, seizures), neuroanatomy, and etiology (congenital and acquired malformations, genetics). Based on different methods and lack of reliability of subtype classification among centers, the SCPE (the previously mentioned European network of population-based surveys and CP registers) adopted a simple classification of 4 CP subtype groups: unilateral spastic, bilateral spastic, dyskinetic, and ataxic. The SCPE participants developed a classification tree[14] and a reference and training manual in CD format that includes video examples of the different clinical patterns of neurologic signs and motor function impairments.[29] Those useful tools have promoted a standardized way of classifying CP subtypes. Groups in other countries, including the United States (Atlanta),[30,31] Western Australia,[32] Quebec, Canada,[33] and South-east Australia,[18] have adopted similar classification systems. Data from these groups have shown similar distributions of CP subtypes.[34] However, work continues toward improving reliability of this classification system.[35] Recent advances in neuroscience and technology, as well as increasing knowledge of age-related features, have led to consideration of broader anatomic features, radiologic findings, causative factors, and timing of injury.[36,37]

International surveillance systems are now using formalized methods to assess function in addition to impairment. The Gross Motor Function Measurement Scale (GMFMS, 88 or 66 items) was developed for clinical use, reduced to a 5-point scale for epidemiologic purposes, The Gross Motor Function Classification System (GMFCS)[38] and extended and revised in 2007. More recently, similar scales for fine motor abilities have been developed: the Manual Ability Classification System (MACS) and the Bimanual Fine Motor Function (BFMF) scales. GMFCS and MACS have been validated and are available online.[39,40] BFMF takes into account asymmetry and allows data to be extracted from medical records. Comparability of results across monitoring programs is greatly facilitated by the use of these measures. Cans and colleagues[34] compared surveillance data reported by groups in Southeast Australia, Norway, Sweden, and France. In the studies reviewed, the proportion of more severely impaired children (level IV/V) on either the GMFCS or BFMF was around 25% to 35% of all CP case children. They found the dyskinetic group to have the highest variability between study sites, which not surprisingly suggests difficulties in classifying mixed types and lower frequencies of dyskinetic CP.

METHODOLOGY

Researchers have employed a variety of methods to measure the frequency of CP in the population. This frequency is measured as prevalence, which is the proportion of the number of individuals with CP among a defined population with CP at a specified period in time. In the United States, there are 5 predominant methods for obtaining prevalence data: (1) notification (reportable disease surveillance); (2) disease registries; (3) periodic population-based surveys; (4) secondary use of administrative data systems; and (5) ongoing, population-based record review.[41] Each data collection mechanism has a different primary purpose, which for most is not estimation of CP prevalence. Therefore, although all systems provide useful information, there are strengths and limitations to each as they pertain to obtaining a complete count of the number of children with CP in a defined community at a specified period in time.

Notification (Reportable Disease Surveillance)

In the United States, all states have laws that require the reporting of selected infectious diseases to the local, district, or state health department. These passive, provider-based reporting systems rely on the receipt of individual case reports from physicians, laboratories, and health care providers, and are simple and nonburdensome. Sometimes developmental disabilities such as CP are also included in such systems. One example is the Georgia Birth Defects Reporting and Information System (GBDRIS), which provides information to the Georgia Department of Human Resources on the incidence, prevalence, trends, and epidemiology of birth defects and related conditions in children from birth to age 6 years. CP is one of the conditions monitored. Because CP is often diagnosed after birth by medical providers in a variety of health care settings, it is not easily captured through a notifiable disease-reporting system such as the GBDRIS, which relies primarily on birth hospitals for case identification.

Disease Registries

Disease registries rely on the voluntary reporting of individuals with specific diseases and are usually based on service provision. Because disease registries are often clinic based, children who do not visit the participating clinics would not be counted in any prevalence estimates produced through analysis of registry data. As a result, disease registries may not be representative of a population.

Periodic Population-based Surveys

Periodic population-based surveys involve the systematic collection of information using a standardized data collection instrument administered as an in-person interview, self-completed questionnaire, or by telephone, or mail. In the United States, The Centers for Disease Control and Prevention's (CDC), The National Center for Health Statistics (NCHS), administers the National Health Interview Survey (NHIS) which includes a Disability Supplement (1994–1995) and Sample Child File (1997–2006) that provide information related to participants' experiences with children and disability. Another NCHS population-based survey that provides valuable information related to developmental disabilities is the State and Local Area Integrated Telephone Survey (SLAITS), which includes the National Survey on Children with Special Health Care Needs (2001). These surveys are conducted using a large sample size and as such are believed to be representative of national characteristics. In addition, these surveys are often more timely than other active methods of data collection. The Sample Child File, for example, is produced annually. Nevertheless, administration of population-based surveys can be labor intensive and costly. Moreover, the collection of data through parental or guardian report is subject to recall bias (that is, differences in accuracy or completeness of reporting information on risk factors and behaviors, due to disparities in recall of past events or experiences between individuals with a diagnosis compared to those without such a diagnosis) and selection bias (differences in the characteristics between individuals participating in a study and those who are not). A further limitation of these surveys that may be particularly important for a population affected by developmental disabilities is that no data are collected for individuals who live in a residential treatment facility or institution.

Secondary Use of Administrative Data

Many administrative data systems with individual-level data can be used for the public health surveillance of developmental disabilities. The most common of these include hospital discharge data, health insurance and Medicaid billing data, and managed-care encounter data. Because these systems are not designed for public health surveillance, the accuracy and completeness of diagnostic information may be uncertain. Other administrative data systems rely on the use of existing aggregate rather than individual-level data. These passive surveillance systems examine federal-, state-, and county-level data for individuals receiving education or diagnostic and treatment services. One example in the United States is the Office of Special Education Programs (OSEP) Annual Reports to Congress on the Implementation of the Individuals with Disabilities Education Act (IDEA). This provider-based reporting mechanism relies on receipt of aggregate reports from each school district in the United States. This type of data collection method is simple, timely, and not burdensome. However, the system may underestimate the population prevalence because not all children with disabilities receive special education services through the school system. Prevalence estimates for some disabilities such as intellectual disabilities can be obtained using OSEP data because there are specific special education exceptionalities for these disabilities. However, it is not possible to describe the special education services of children with CP or measure prevalence of CP using OSEP Annual Reports for several reasons: (1) the program area in which significant numbers of children with CP are served (ie, orthopedic impairment) also includes children with other motor disorders; (2) many children with CP receive services under the other health impairment exceptionality, which is a program area for children with other medical conditions as well; (3) those with co-occurring intellectual disability (ID) are most often served through an ID exceptionality.

Ongoing, Population-based Record Review

Ongoing, population-based record review is an active surveillance system whereby information is systematically collected on individual children by standardized data collection instruments through review of existing records at administrative data sources. Programs using this method track the number of children identified with CP using multiple sources in the community that diagnose, treat, or serve children with developmental disabilities. Examples of this type of data collection include the CP surveillance programs in the United States and internationally. In the United States, the ADDM Network, funded by the Centers for Disease Control and Prevention, currently conducts surveillance of CP and other developmental disabilities in 4 communities. SCPE and the Australia Cerebral Palsy Register, which is comprised of numerous registers for CP surveillance across Australia, conduct record reviews and receive notification of CP cases from other reporting sources.

For this type of surveillance, participants do not need to be contacted as a part of data collection, so there is minimal burden on families affected by CP. Objective reliable methods for determining surveillance case definition are established, and extensive training and quality control measures are implemented to ensure adherence to data collection and case determination guidelines and reliable resultant prevalence estimates. Many of the surveillance programs that employ population-based record review do not depend solely on previously documented CP diagnoses to identify children, as descriptions of motor findings consistent with CP are also used to determine case status. Incorporating information from multiple health, education, and service providers rather than relying on only one facility or one type of facility to identify children allows for more complete coverage for case identification in a defined population. Because individual-level data are collected, the identified case series may also be used to address future research questions and may be linked to other databases such as birth certificate files and census data, providing even more information about individuals with CP. The surveillance programs in the United States, Europe, and Australia have been ongoing for many decades, thus affording the ability to examine prevalence estimates of CP in the same population and using the same methods for classifying CP over time. The ADDM Network is strengthened by its heterogeneous population characteristics that enable examination of various racial/ethnic subgroups.

Although this method provides a reasonably complete picture of the population affected by CP, there are some limitations. Because this is an active surveillance method using multiple sources, it is more labor and time intensive and costly to operate than most passive systems. For the ADDM Network, in particular, which relies solely on records, information within the system is dependent on the availability and quality of these records. Some of the records may not contain the necessary information to confirm case status because the system relies on information that has been collected for purposes other than public health surveillance. For the system in the United States, the prevalence of children with mild CP may be underestimated, because these children may not have come to the attention of service providers in early childhood and records of children in regular education, in private schools, or who are being home-schooled are not reviewed. Nevertheless, data from the ADDM Network indicate that these exceptions likely represent a very small proportion of children with CP.[31]

PREVALENCE

Prevalence is calculated as a proportion, and careful attention is necessary when measuring the numerator and choosing the corresponding population denominator. The international community of epidemiologists, who conduct surveillance of CP, grapples with many of the same methodological issues in obtaining population-based CP prevalence estimates. Issues related to obtaining an accurate numerator include the definition of inclusion and exclusion criteria for case determination, evaluation of completeness of case ascertainment, comparison of prevalence and trends, and ensuring validity. To make appropriate comparisons across surveillance systems and over time, it is imperative that the details of these issues are well understood.

There are 5 main CP inclusion and exclusion criteria areas that differ across surveillance systems. These areas include (1) the minimum age of survival, (2) hypotonia, (3) severity, (4) postneonatally acquired CP and timing of the injury, and (5) select chromosomal anomalies, genetic syndromes, metabolic diseases, and mitochondrial disorders. A survey of international surveillance systems and registers provided data on the characteristics of these programs.[42] Approximately half of the international surveillance registers do not have a minimum age of survival for inclusion as a CP case. Of those registers that do impose a minimum age criterion, there is considerable variation from 1 to 8 years of age. With respect to severity, many systems do not apply severity criteria to determine case inclusion. Of those that do, often a combination of neurologic signs, dysfunction, motor impairment by age 5 years, or Level 1 on the GMFCS is applied. Most surveillance programs do not include hypotonic CP. Data from the ADDM Network, which does include hypotonic CP cases in its monitoring efforts, found only 2.6% of cases had hypotonic CP.[31] The overwhelming majority of CP registers includes postneonatally acquired CP cases and has the ability to exclude these children for specific analyses. Of the programs that define a maximum age of cerebral damage, the age varies from 2 to 8 years. Two set of criteria currently exist detailing the specific chromosomal anomalies, genetic syndromes, and metabolic and mitochondrial disorders that constitute CP. Many of the current surveillance programs operationalize the Badawi[17] or SCPE[14] criteria.

All surveillance programs are faced with the challenge of attaining complete ascertainment of all children with CP within a specified geographic area at a specific period in time. From the perspective of birth prevalence, one issue influencing under ascertainment is migration from the surveillance area between birth and age of identification. If it is not possible to follow the entire birth cohort to determine the CP status at the defined age, then birth prevalence will be an underestimate of the "true prevalence" because a proportion of CP cases migrate beyond geographic ascertainment. Another challenge for ascertainment is the type of source for data collection. Three sites in the ADDM Network, which relies on multiple source record review, do not have access to education records, rather only records from clinical and service providers. Although data from the Metropolitan Atlanta Developmental Disability Surveillance Program (MADDSP), one of the ADDM Network sites, indicate that prevalence of CP is not significantly affected by under ascertainment of CP cases identified uniquely from special education sources, prevalences reported from the other three sites is likely an underestimate. MADDSP can only review records of children receiving public education and therefore may miss children who are in private school or are being home-schooled. As previously mentioned, this is believed to be a small proportion of CP cases (because many are identified through clinical sources) but still remains a source of under ascertainment.

The same rigor that is applied when ascertaining the number of individuals with CP in a specified population must also be used to choose an appropriate denominator for calculation of prevalence. The most common denominator used to report CP prevalence is live births. Many CP registers also report prevalence using neonatal survivors as the denominator. Live birth and neonatal survivor denominator data are useful when examining etiologic questions. It can be argued that neonatal survivors are the more appropriate denominator as neonatal deaths do not have the potential to be ascertained as CP cases. Use of neonatal survivors is particularly important when examining CP prevalence by birth weight (BW) or gestational age, as infants of extremely low birth weight (ELBW, <1000g) very low birth weight (VLBW <1500g) or preterm birth (< 37 weeks gestation) have a higher neonatal mortality rate than those of greater birth weights or gestational ages. Therefore, at lower birth weights and earlier gestational ages, the effect of using these 2 different denominators can be significant. Paneth and colleagues[43] stipulate that using live births as the denominator for lower birth weight groups is the only means of obtaining a picture of the net contribution of improving survival to the population prevalence of CP. The choice of denominator is one that differs across registers, most often due to ease of availability of vital statistics data. Nevertheless, the denominator must be taken into consideration when comparing prevalence across studies. A handful of surveillance programs use children as the denominator to calculate period prevalence. These data are most informative for service provision and planning. Due to differences across CP surveillance programs with respect to the aforementioned methodological issues, it is crucial that each program assess the comparability of their own program's methods over time and account for any within-program methodological changes before examining trends. Once internal validity is established, comparison of trends across CP surveillance programs is appropriate.

Across the various surveillance programs in developed countries, estimates of CP prevalence overall using live births and neonatal survivors have been comparable, most estimates being 2.0 per 1000 (**Table 1**). Estimates using children as the denominator have been somewhat higher, ranging from 3.1 to 4.4 per 1000. Among population-based studies of CP, males have been found to have a higher prevalence of CP than females, with sex ratios ranging from 1.1:1 to 1.5:1.[31,44,45] Although there have been few studies that examined racial/ethnic differences in prevalence, a higher prevalence in black non-Hispanic children compared with white non-Hispanic children has

Table 1
Prevalence of CP per 1000 live births, neonatal survivors, or children from select epidemiologic studies, 2000 onward

Reference	Location	Study Population	Birth Cohorts[a]	Overall Prevalence			
				N	Denominator	Prevalence	95% CI
Colver et al, 2000[55]	North east England	4–10-year-olds	1989–1993	117	47, 691	2.5[c]	2.0, 2.9
Hagberg B et al, 2001[63]	Western Sweden	At least 4 years	1991–1994	241	113, 724	2.1[b]	1.9, 2.4
Parkes et al, 2001[51]	Northern Ireland	5-year-olds	1981–1993	784	NR	2.2[b]	2.1, 2.4
Nordmark et al, 2001[119]	Southern Sweden	5–8-year-olds	1990–1993	145	65, 514	2.2[b]	1.9, 2.6
Topp et al, 2001[52]	Eastern Denmark	At least 4 years	1987–1990	299	NR	2.4[b]	NR
SCPE, 2002[54]	11 European centres	At least 4 years	1980–1990	NR	NR	2.1[c]	2.0, 2.1
Winter et al, 2002[30]	Metropolitan Atlanta, GA, USA	0-year-olds	1986–1991	443	216, 471	2.0[c]	1.9, 2.2
Himmelmann et al, 2005[48]	Western Sweden	At least 4 years	1995–1998	170	88, 371	1.9[b]	1.7, 2.2
Sundrum et al, 2005[120]	United Kingdom	At least 2 years	1982–1997	293	105, 760	2.8[b]	NR
Bhasin et al, 2006[45]	Metropolitan Atlanta, GA, USA	8-year-olds	1992	135	43, 593	3.1[d]	2.6, 3.7
Serdaroglu et al, 2006[121]	Turkey	2–16-year-olds	1996	186	41, 861	4.4[d]	3.8, 5.1
Watson et al, 2009[122]	Western Australia	At least 5 years	1995–1999	303	126, 681	2.4[c]	2.1, 2.7
Yeargin-Allsopp et al, 2008[31]	Metropolitan Atlanta, GA, USA	8-year-olds	1994	416	114, 897	3.6[d]	3.3, 4.0
Andersen GL et al, 2008[123]	Norway	Birth–4 years	1996–1998	374	NR	2.1[b]	NR
Ameson C et al, 2009[1]	3 United States communities	8-year-olds	1996	227	68, 272	3.3[d]	2.9, 3.8

[a] Most recent birth cohort(s)/time period is reported.
[b] Live birth as denominator.
[c] Neonatal survivor as denominator.
[d] Children as denominator.
Abbreviations: CI, confidence interval; NR, not reported; Prev, prevalence.

been reported for 3 time periods in metropolitan Atlanta and overall from the 3 CDC ADDM Network sites in 2002.[31,44,46,47] Among all studies of CP, spastic subtypes have been found to be more common, with fewer percentages of the ataxic and dyskinetic subtypes.[30,31,46,48] Little is known currently about the prevalence of CP in developing countries. Whereas differences in reported prevalence may reflect accurate differences in population prevalence, variations may also reflect differences in the methodology of both the numerator and denominator. Efforts are being made to foster international communication to understand these variations and strive for comparability where possible. One of the greatest strengths of the numerous surveillance registers in existence is that they have been in operation for many decades, which affords the opportunity to examine trends in CP prevalence over time.

Neonatal intensive care practices have experienced a dramatic evolution over the past 3 decades and these changes have had significant effects on infant mortality and morbidity. The early 1980s were marked by use of enhanced assisted ventilation; the 1990s brought the introduction and widespread use of surfactant and antenatal and postnatal steroid therapies. The American Academy of Pediatrics 2002 recommendations brought yet another practice shift, with decreased postnatal corticosteroid use and emphasis on sepsis prevention methods.[49,50] In many areas, the overall prevalence of CP has been stable over time.[30,51] In other areas, overall CP prevalence has varied. For birth years 1987 through 1998, Western Sweden found a significant decline in their total CP prevalence.[48] In Denmark, Topp and colleagues[52] also found a significant decreasing trend in overall CP birth prevalence from their 2 most recent time periods; 3.0 in 1983 through 1986 to 2.4 in 1987 through 1990. When data from the SCPE Network were harmonized, they found that an overall upward trend in the late 1970s was followed by a plateau in the 1980s and a nonsignificant downward trend toward 1990 in the overall prevalence of CP.[53,54] To the contrary, data from north-east England from 1964 through 1993 indicated a consistent upward trend from 1.7 per 1000 neonatal survivors in 1964 through 1968 to 2.5 per 1000 neonatal survivors in 1989 through 1993.[55] Nevertheless, all surveillance programs have experienced substantial prevalence changes over time within various risk factor subgroups, such as among those born with ELBW (<1000 g) and VLBW (<1500 g), or very preterm (< 32 weeks).

CAUSES AND RISK FACTORS

A plethora of research has been conducted on the causes and risk factors of CP, most of which indicates that the causal pathways may be numerous and the etiology multifactorial. Examination of risk factors is commonly categorized by the timing of their proposed occurrence: prenatal, perinatal, and postnatal. Prenatal and perinatal risk factors include ELBW and VLBW, preterm birth, neonatal encephalopathy, multiple pregnancy, assisted reproductive technology, infection and inflammation, and genetic factors. Prevention of postnatal causes holds the most promise for decreasing the prevalence of CP.

Birth Weight and Gestational Age

The inverse relationship between increased risk of CP and being born at lower birth weights or earlier gestational ages, or both, has been consistently well supported over time (**Table 2**). Population-based surveillance data indicate that the prevalence of CP among VLBW children ranges from 51 to 73 per 1000 neonatal survivors, and is lowest (1–2 per 1000 neonatal survivors) and most reflective of overall prevalence for children born at normal birth weight (NBW) (≥2500 g). Similar results, in terms of

Table 2
Prevalence of CP per 1000 live births or neonatal survivors by birth weight or gestational age from select epidemiologic studies, 2000 onward

Reference	Location	Birth Cohorts[a]	N	Birth Prevalence								
				Overall		<1500 g		1500–2499 g		≥2500 g		
				Prev	95% CI	Prev	95% CI	Prev	95% CI	Prev	95% CI	
SCPE, 2002[54]	7 Centres in Europe	1980–1990[d]	3444	2.1[b]	2.0, 2.2	72.5	67.5, 77.7	11.1	10.4, 11.8	1.1	1.1, 1.2	
Winter et al, 2002[30]	Metropolitan Atlanta, Georgia	1986–1991	443	2.0[b]	1.9, 2.2	59.5	50.3, 69.6	6.2	5.0, 7.7	1.1	0.9, 1.2	
Himmelman et al, 2005[48]	Western Sweden	1995–1998	170	1.9[c]	1.7, 2.2	63.4	46.2, 87.2	6.7	4.4, 10.2	1.2	1.0, 1.5	
Watson et al, 2009[122]	Western Australia	1995–1999	303	2.4[b]	2.1, 2.7	50.7	37.8, 63.6	8.3	6.1, 10.5	1.6	1.4, 1.9	

Reference	Location	Birth Cohorts[a]	N	Overall		28–31 weeks		32–36 weeks		≥37 weeks	
				Prev	95% CI	Prev	95% CI	Prev	95% CI	Prev	95% CI
SCPE, 2002[54]	7 Centres in Europe	1980–1990[d]	3444	2.1[b]	2.0, 2.2	79.5	73.3, 86.0	8.0	7.2, 8.8	1.2	1.1, 1.2
Himmelman et al, 2005[48]	Western Sweden	1995–1998	170	1.9[c]	1.7, 2.2	50.1	36.6, 68.6	6.7	4.7, 9.5	1.1	0.9, 1.4
Watson et al, 2009[122]	Western Australia	1995–1999	303	2.4[b]	2.1, 2.7	35.0	26.5, 43.5	4.9	3.4, 6.4	1.7	1.5, 1.9

[a] Most recent birth cohort(s)/time period is reported.
[b] Neonatal survivors as denominator.
[c] Live births as denominator.
[d] Birth cohorts across centers vary.
Abbreviations: CI, confidence interval; Prev, prevalence.

magnitude and differential birth weight risk, are found when examining very preterm, preterm, and term deliveries. While birth weight is more commonly used in epidemiologic analyses to evaluate trends in CP prevalence than gestational age, this is more often attributable to completeness of vital statistics data on birth weight than to implications that this is a more scientifically valid metric.

The effects of neonatal intensive care improvements over time, which differ by birth weight and gestational age, have particular implications for infants born at ELBW (<1000 g) and extremely (< 28 weeks) and very preterm birth (28 - 31 weeks). Data from Cleveland, Ohio, in the United States on the neurodevelopmental outcomes among ELBW children found that survival increased from 49% to 71% from the early 1980s through early 2000s, yet the proportion of ELBW children with CP rose from the early 1980s through 1990s from 8% to 13%, respectively, and then decreased to 5% during the period from 2000 through 2002.[50] Data from eastern Denmark found that the overall significant decline in CP prevalence through the 1980s was driven by a significant decrease among children with CP born very preterm (≤31 weeks).[52] Similarly in the Province of Alberta, Canada, the steep increase in CP prevalence among extremely preterm births peaked in 1992 through 1994 at 131 per 1000 live births and fell to 19 per 1000 live births by 2001 through 2003.[56] Himmelman and colleagues[48] found that in Western Sweden the rising trend among the extremely preterm group in the 1980s stabilized in the early 1990s; this was followed by decreases in the prevalence of CP among children born very preterm, moderately preterm, and term, the latter 2 being statistically significant. Similar results in the association over time between CP and gestational age were found by the Western Australia register.[57] For both systems, in the 1990s the previously similar rates among extremely and very preterm births began to change with the CP prevalence among the extremely preterm group approximately double that of the very preterm group by the late 1990s. Demonstrating geographic differences in the effect of improved neonatal care, Doyle and colleagues[58] found that in Victoria, Australia, the prevalence of CP among ELBW children did not significantly change over 3 cross-sectional equal eras spanning 1979 through 1992, and data from Nova Scotia and North-east England showed a significant increase in prevalence among very preterm infants from 1993 through 2002 and 1970 through 1994, respectively.[59,60]

For VLBW infants (<1500 g), the SCPE Network found that from 1980 through 1996 there was a significant decrease in the prevalence of CP from 60.6 per 1000 live births to 39.5 per 1000 live births for this birth weight group. This significant decline was restricted to children born weighing 1000 through 1499 g and although the point estimates were higher, this trend held true when neonatal survivor denominator data were used.[61] In addition to the previously noted studies on ELBW and preterm birth, These data demonstrate that infants born at less than 1500 g have both a better chance of survival and of not having a severe neurologic motor impairment. The data previously discussed from Cleveland, Ohio, on ELBW infants reported consistent findings for ELBW infants born during the period 2000 through 2002.[50] These data are encouraging. Nevertheless, it is crucial to highlight the continued importance of preventing preterm delivery and VLBW.

Whereas children born with ELBW and VLBW are clearly at greatest risk for CP, more than half of CP cases occurs among infants born at NBW, term, or near-term. Throughout the 1980s and 1990s, there was no apparent decrease in CP prevalence among term infants. Over these time frames, studies have elucidated a handful of causes for CP in term and near-term children, such as intrauterine exposure to infection and coagulation disorders, which point to the potential for prevention.[62] Post-term delivery (>41 weeks) is also a risk factor for CP, reportedly 3 times that of term birth.[16]

Small sample sizes among cohorts of children with CP born at lower birth weights make examination of the characteristics and subtypes of these children challenging. However, a handful of population-based studies have been able to investigate these issues. The decreased trend in the SCPE Network's reports of CP prevalence related to a reduction in frequency of bilateral spastic CP among infants of birth weight 1000g to 1499g, spastic CP for those with birth weight less than 1500 g was predominantly caused by periventricular lesions. Periventricular leukomalacia damages bilateral motor tracts in most cases, leading to bilateral spastic cerebral palsy, whereas periventricular hemorrhage leads to mainly unilateral motor-tract damage and unilateral spastic cerebral palsy. The prevalence data here suggest a decline mainly of periventricular leukomalacia in children of birth weight less than 1500 g. The other subtype that has been examined with respect to birth weight and gestational age is dyskinetic CP. Dyskinetic CP was found to be more common in term newborns compared with those born prematurely. Data from western Sweden found an increase in the prevalence of dyskinetic CP in term newborns from 1983 through 1998.[48,63,64]

Neonatal Encephalopathy

Badawi and colleagues[65] linked the population-based Western Australian case controlled study of a newborn encephalopathy cohort to the Western Australia Cerebral Palsy Register. These investigators compared the characteristics among children whose CP followed newborn encephalopathy with those with CP following an uncomplicated neonatal course. Intrapartum causes of CP were found to be uncommon. Among term infants, only 24% of CP case infants followed newborn encephalopathy, whereas 76% of cases had been normal during the newborn period. Following term encephalopathy, 13% of infants with moderate to severe encephalopathy developed CP. The highest rate was among those with neonatal seizures. Those with term encephalopathy and CP were more likely to have a severe, spastic quadriplegic or dyskinetic subtype, and were 4 times more likely to die during the period from diagnosis through 6 years of age.

Multiple Pregnancy

CP occurs more commonly among multiple births. In the Epipage Study, Bonellie and colleagues[66] used a Scottish register for 1984 through 1990 to examine etiologic factors and patterns of CP among multiple and singleton births. This study found twins to be 4.8 times more likely to develop CP than singletons. Being a twin was found to carry an increased risk of CP independent of prematurity and birth weight. Looking at birth weight for gestational age, twins had from 3.5 to 5.5 times higher rates of CP in all quintiles of birth weight, the greatest variance being in the lowest quintile. Death of a co-twin increased the rate of CP by a factor of 6 compared with when both twins were live-born. Twins were more likely to develop spastic quadriplegia, whereas singletons were more likely to develop dyskinetic or ataxic CP. Birth order had no effect on the rate of CP. Discordance of at least 30% was associated with a 5-fold greater risk of CP, equally distributed between the larger and smaller twin. Pregnancy complications (such as growth restriction) were not associated with CP among twins over and above the risk from preterm birth itself. The rate of CP associated with delivery preterm of a growth-restricted infant was lower than for other causes of preterm delivery, perhaps because such delivery is often by elective cesarean section avoiding the inflammatory risks of labor.

Assisted Reproduction

Reproductive technologies are emerging rapidly, as a result, their possible association with developmental outcomes is an area of wide interest. Several studies from

Denmark have provided information on such associations. Lidegaard and colleagues[67] demonstrated a statistically significant 80% increase in CP among singleton children conceived by in vitro fertilization (IVF). Pinborg and colleagues[68] compared outcomes of twins and singletons conceived by assisted reproductive technologies (ART) and naturally conceived twins. They cross-linked the national medical birth registry, the In Vitro Fertilization Register, National Patients' Register, and the Danish Psychiatric Central Register to examine outcomes of conceptions that occurred during the period 1995 through 2000. Twins conceived using ARTs had a similar risk of neurologic sequelae as naturally conceived twins and singletons conceived using ARTs.

Hvidtjorn and colleagues[69] published a population-based cohort study, that included all live-born singletons and twins born in Denmark from January 1, 1995 through December 31, 2000. Children conceived with in vitro fertilization (9,255 children) were identified through the In Vitro Fertilization Register; children conceived without in vitro fertilization (394,713 children) were identified through the Danish Medical Birth Registry. CP diagnoses were obtained from the National Register of Hospital Discharges. This group found that it was the increased proportions of preterm deliveries following IVF for twins and singletons that were associated with the increased risk of CP. The independent effect of in vitro fertilization vanished after additional adjustment for multiplicity or preterm delivery.

Infection and Inflammation

The role of infection and inflammation in the etiology of preterm birth has gained prominence in recent years.[70] It is known that preterm infants have higher rates of exposure to ascending intrauterine infection. The prevalence of positive amniotic fluid cultures and raised amniotic fluid cytokines remains high in women who have labor earlier than 34 weeks, regardless of low rates of bacterial vaginosis, chorioamnionitis, and urinary infection in pregnancy.[71] It remains unclear whether cytokines can cross the placenta and how much of the measured fetal load is of maternal origin. It has been suggested that cytokines measured in maternal or fetal compartments reflect local inflammation.[72]

Nelson and colleagues[73] examined DNA extracted from archived blood samples from very preterm infants with CP and matched controls. These investigators looked for the presence of single nucleotide polymorphisms in proteins associated with nitric oxide production, thrombosis or thromboprophylaxis, hypertension, and inflammation. Genotypic frequencies in several of the tested variants were differentially distributed in children with CP and controls. These variations in genetic coding may affect protein function/interaction, altering the balance between inflammation and suppression.

Graham and colleagues[74] performed a retrospective case-control study over a 7-year period of birth (1994–2001) of births of 23 through 34 weeks' gestation with white matter lesions and gestational age-matched controls. Severe intrapartum hypoxia/ischemia was found to be a rare association with white matter injury in this preterm group. Case infants had significantly higher rates of positive cultures of blood, cerebrospinal fluid, and tracheal fluid than control infants. Chorioamnionitis and funisitis were not associated histologically with white matter injury. These results suggest that multiple insults converge on cytokine production as a final common pathway to central nervous system injury. Some insults cause direct damage; other insults prime the immune system, making the fetal brain more vulnerable.

Several investigators have theorized a stepwise pathway of sensitization followed by injury, so that mild hypoxia may be damaging if the baby's compensatory mechanisms have been downregulated or disabled by another inflammatory insult.[75–77]

Genetics

An increasing body of evidence points to strong genetic influences on the occurrence of CP, and a multifactorial inheritance pattern is suggested. This evidence implies etiologic and genetic heterogeneity with complex interactions, and multiple environmental influences.[78] There are multiple points along a causal path for cerebral palsy that may be vulnerable to genetic variations. Single nucleotide polymorphisms and thrombophilias provide examples.

Single nucleotide polymorphisms in proteins are associated with the *inflammatory* process (eg, nitric oxide production, thrombosis or thromboprophylaxis, hypertension, and inflammation). Variations in the genetic coding may affect protein function or interaction, altering the balance between inflammation and suppression.[70]

The coagulation cascade is the body's response to a breach in the vascular system and is part of the body's hemostatic mechanism. The coagulation cascade normally is balanced by procoagulation and anticoagulation mechanisms. However, there are instances in which this balance is altered to favor either procoagulation or anticoagulation. Thrombophilia favors procoagulation and is an inherited or acquired condition that predisposes individuals to thromboembolism. Common inherited thrombophilias include mutations in factor V Leiden, polymorphisms in the gene for 5,10-methylenetetrahydrofolate reductase (MTHFR) associated with hyperhomocysteinemia, and mutations in the plasminogen activator inhibitor-1 (PAI-1) gene.[79–81]

Most thrombophilias require another risk factor to express the adverse phenotype. In pregnancy the overall homeostatic balance is already altered toward hypercoagulability. The presence of inflammatory cytokines (perhaps upregulated in response to infection) in conjunction with an inherited thrombophilia may provoke the development of thrombosis. Thromboses as well as inflammation have been implicated as important factors in the causal pathway of CP.[81]

A group from South Australia[80] performed a population-based, large case-control study to investigate associations between CP and hereditary thrombophilias. These investigators compared the prevalence of thrombophilic polymorphisms, common in white populations, in different types of CP cases at different gestational ages and in controls. Genomic DNA from newborn screening cards of 443 white CP case infants and 883 white control infants was tested for factor V Leiden (FVL, G1691A), prothrombin gene mutation (PGM, G20210A), and 2 single base mutations of methylenetetrahydrofolate reductase (MTHFR C677T and MTHFR A1298C). Term CP was not associated with any of these thrombophilias. FVL and PGM were not found to be associated with CP when they existed alone. MTHFR C677T (homo- or heterozygous) was associated with a significant increased risk of diplegia, especially earlier than 32 weeks. MTHFR A1298C (homozygous) was negatively associated with quadriplegia (odds ratio 0.33 [CI 0.1–0.87]). Combinations of thrombophilias had additive effects.

Genetic variations play a role in the complex interrelationship involving inflammation, coagulation, control of blood flow, and function of vascular endothelium in placenta and brain. Maternal and pregnancy conditions such as preterm birth, placental abruption, preeclampsia, and chorioamnionitis are affected. Environmental factors interact with genetic characteristics to produce risk.[82]

ASSOCIATED IMPAIRMENTS AND CONDITIONS

The defining motor impairments of CP are often accompanied by cognitive, behavioral, and sensory impairments, as well as epilepsy. Data from population-based studies have reported the proportion of children with CP with co-occurring impairments to range from 31% to 65% for intellectual disability (IQ <70), 20% to

46% for epilepsy, 2% to 6% for hearing loss, and 2% to 19% for vision impairment (**Table 3**). The 2 studies that examined speech and language deficits as associated conditions showed that 28% to 43% of children with CP have this co-occurring condition. The MADDSP in Atlanta, the only surveillance system to monitor autism spectrum disorders (ASDs) in addition to CP, found that 9% of children with CP had an ASD. The severity of the associated impairments often has a profound impact on the ability to assess impairments, management, functional attainment, and life expectancy. Therefore, differential classification of CP must be accompanied by information about not only the core but also the associated impairments.

Cognitive Impairment

More than half of individuals with CP have some type of intellectual or neuropsychological impairment; however, there is not a definitive or absolute correlation between the degree of intellectual impairment and the type or subclass of CP.[83] The severity of spastic motor impairment does correlate with the degree of cognitive deficit. Those with spastic quadriplegia have the highest risk of cognitive impairment and those with spastic hemiplegia the lowest. This finding is in contrast to dyskinetic types, wherein this relationship is not present.[84] There is also a strong association between greater intellectual impairment in children with CP and the presence of epilepsy, an abnormal electroencephalogram (EEG), or an abnormal neuroimaging study.[85]

There are clearly exceptions, and it is crucial that persons with significant physical involvement be afforded the opportunity to demonstrate their mental abilities. Children with different forms of CP may be difficult to assess because of the motor deficits, and in some forms of CP (eg, spastic diplegia) the differences between performance and verbal intelligence test scores actually increase with age.[86] Nonverbal learning impairments, with relative weaknesses in visual-spatial abilities, are common.[87,88] The proportion of children with CP and without severe associated impairment has been reported to vary from one third to one half depending on CP type and birth weight.[34] About 40% of children with hemiplegia have normal cognitive abilities, whereas most children with tetraplegia are severely cognitively impaired.[83,89] There is no association between cognitive level and location of brain damage (left or right).[90]

The impact of associated cognitive impairment must be considered when informing parents about their child's prognosis. Severe intellectual impairment, for example, has a strong influence on walking ability in children with unilateral spastic CP.[91] In addition, children with cerebral palsy and intellectual disability are more likely to experience emotional and behavioral symptoms.[92]

Speech impairment, including dysarthria and aphasia, is common and strongly associated with the type and severity of motor involvement. For example, articulation disorders and impaired speech intelligibility are present in 38% of children with CP. Language (as opposed to speech) deficits in CP correlate with intellectual limitations.[93]

Epilepsy

Odding and colleagues[83] reported that between 22% to 40% of people with cerebral palsy have epilepsy, with the prevalence varying by subtype. Epilepsy was reported in 28% to 35% of children with hemiplegic CP, 19% to 36% with tetraplegic CP, 14% with diplegic CP, 13% to 16% with ataxic CP, and 8% to 13% with dyskinetic CP. These results are consistent with those of other studies.[93] Epilepsy is most prevalent in quadriplegia (50%–94%), followed by hemiplegia and tetraplegia. Higher prevalence is also associated with more severe disability. Among those with severe cognitive impairment, 94% have epilepsy.[89] Children with CP and epilepsy tend to have a more severe epilepsy course. Studies have shown children with CP to have a higher

Table 3
Proportion of children with cerebral palsy with co-occurring developmental disabilities

Study	Study Population	Study Year(s)	Intellectual Disability	Proportion of Children with CP with Co-Occurring Condition				
				Epilepsy	Hearing Loss	Vision Impairment	Autism Spectrum Disorders	Speech and Language
Van Naarden Braun K, Doernberg N, Yeargin-Allsopp M, personal communication; 2009	8-year-olds	2006	43[a]	43	6	16	9	-
Murphy et al[44]	10-year-olds	1985–1987	65[a]	46	4	10	-	-
Watson et al[122]	Birth to 5 years	1995–1999	37[a]	32	4	2	-	-
Himmelmann et al[124]	4–8 years	1991–1998	40[a]	33	-	19	-	-
Beckung E. et al[125]	8–12 years	1991–1997	52[a]	21	2	7	-	43
Surveillance of Cerebral Palsy in Europe (SCPE)[55]	At least 4 years	1980–1990	31[b]	21	-	11	-	-
Andersen GL et al[123]	At least 4 years	1996–1998	31[a]	28	4	5	-	28
Parks J et al[51]	Birth to 5 years	1981–1993	41[a]	20	2	10	-	-

[a] IQ <70.
[b] IQ <50.

incidence of epilepsy with onset within the first year of age (47% versus 10%), history of neonatal seizures (19% versus 3%), status epilepticus (16% versus 1.7%), need for polytherapy (25% versus 3%), and treatment with second-line antiepileptic drugs (31% versus 6.7%). Generalized and partial epilepsy are predominant.[85,93]

Sensory Impairment

The etiologies of diplegic and hemiplegic CP commonly involve pathology of the central nervous system that alters normal development of the somatosensory system.[94,95] Deficits in stereognosis and 2-point discrimination have been found in 44% to 51% of all children with cerebral palsy, with term children most severely impacted.[96] Sensory impairments are most common among those with hemiplegia, in whom 90% have significant bilateral sensory deficits. Stereognosis and proprioception are the chief modalities affected bilaterally. The degree of sensory impairment does not correlate with the degree of motor impairment.[97] Bilateral tactile deficits are common in bilateral spastic (diplegic) and unilateral spastic (hemiplegic) cerebral palsy subtypes, including those with milder motor involvement.[98]

People with cerebral palsy experience more chronic pain than the general population. Back pain is most prevalent across all types of cerebral palsy. Foot and ankle pain is most prevalent in those with diplegia, knee pain in tetraplegia, and neck and shoulder pain and headache in persons with dyskinesia. Chronic pain has been associated with low life satisfaction and deterioration of functional skills.[99–101]

Visual Impairment and Hearing Loss

Visual defects are common in children with CP. More than 70% of children with cerebral palsy have been found to have low visual acuity.[102] Although there is an increased presence of strabismus, amblyopia, nystagmus, optic atrophy, and refractive errors, central visual impairment seems to contribute significantly to the acuity problems. Children whose CP is due to periventricular leukomalacia are also more likely to have visual perceptual problems.[93] For children with cerebral palsy and a history of prematurity there is a higher prevalence of retinopathy, cortical visual impairment, and strabismus than in those with cerebral palsy without prematurity. There is no difference in refractive error between premature children with or without cerebral palsy.[103] Hearing loss is present in approximately 2% to 6% of children with CP. Significant risk factors include VLBW, kernicterus, neonatal meningitis, severe hypoxic-ischemic insults, intellectual disability, and abnormal neuroimaging.[93]

Feeding, Growth, and Endocrine Problems

Feeding problems are common in cerebral palsy.[104] During the first year of life, 57% of children with cerebral palsy have sucking problems, 38% have swallowing problems, 80% have been fed nonorally on at least one occasion, and more than 90% have clinically significant oral motor dysfunction.[105] Among children with spastic quadriplegia, one third require assisted feeding. More severe functional involvement (a GMFCS Level of IV or V) and microcephaly are associated with the need for assisted feeding.[106] (See also Pruitt and Tsai, this issue).

Linear growth is typically reduced in cerebral palsy. The California Department of Developmental Services looked at percentiles of height and weight of patients with CP over a 15-year period. This group found persons with CP to have height and weight centiles close to those of the general population for the highest functioning groups with CP, but to lag substantially for other groups. Presence of a feeding tube was associated with greater height and weight in the lowest functioning groups, with centiles for weight being 2 to 5 kg higher for those with gastrostomy tubes.[107]

Bone mineral density (BMD) is reduced in adolescents with spastic CP. Femoral osteopenia is present in 75% of all children with moderate to severe cerebral palsy, and in almost all children who cannot stand. Children with severe CP develop clinically significant osteopenia over the course of their lives. Unlike elderly adults, this is not primarily from true losses in bone mineral, but from a rate of growth in bone mineral that is diminished relative to healthy children.[108] Multiple aspects of skeletal growth and development, including skeletal maturation, are frequently altered in children with moderate to severe CP.[109] (See also Houlihan and Stevenson, this issue.)

Urogenital Problems

Children with CP gain bladder and bowel control at older ages compared with their siblings and healthy children, and also have more frequent enuresis and urinary infections.[110] Primary enuresis is present in about 25% of children and adolescents with cerebral palsy. The most important determinants are intellectual ability and tetraplegia.[111] Voiding dysfunction has been reported in more than half of children with cerebral palsy.[112] Urinary symptoms and pathologic urodynamic findings increase along with the degree of motor function impairment shown by the GMFCS. Pathologic urodynamic findings can be found in symptomatic and asymptomatic patients.[113] In one study evaluating children with cerebral palsy referred for daytime enuresis at age 10 years, 85% were found to have abnormal videourodynamics, with treatment leading to improvement.[114]

TRANSITIONING

As children with CP reach young adulthood, supportive services such as rehabilitation, special education, and specialized pediatric care often cease. Without these services, young adults with CP can experience new problems with daily activities or worsening of existing conditions, at a time when most have decreased access to services. The new social roles in young adulthood, coupled with the vulnerabilities exacerbated as a result of declining support systems, underscore the need to understand issues across the life span as children with CP grow into adulthood.

Population-based data on the consequences of CP are limited. In the 1990s, the CDC conducted one such epidemiologic study with a subset of children with CP identified through surveillance activities. This study found that 77% of young adults with CP, identified during childhood, experienced limitations in daily functioning. Also, approximately 50% of young adults with CP, without intellectual disability, hearing loss, vision loss, or epilepsy were competitively employed, compared with 16% of young adults with CP and one of these co-occurring developmental disabilities.[115,116] Data from one of the largest studies examining postsecondary education outcomes uses data from the Department of Education and categorizes children based their special education exceptionality.[117] The utility of these data for CP are limited because not all children with CP are receiving services under the same special education exceptionality. Children with CP in special education receive services under several exceptionalities, often differing by the presence of co-occurring conditions. For example, data show that 73% of children with co-occurring intellectual disability receive services under an intellectual disability exceptionality, compared with children with CP with isolated motor impairment, of whom 37% were served through other health impairment, 28% through orthopedic impairment, and 7% through an intellectual disability exceptionality.[118] Much has changed in the past decade since this work was first conducted on young adults by the CDC. It is important to evaluate the effect of current challenges as well as new and unique opportunities that have become available for individuals with CP, to ensure that individuals with CP have a full range of life options. (See also Riehle and Rutkowski, this issue.)

SUMMARY

Although the definition of CP, the most common motor disability of childhood, has been reexamined in recent years, the core components remain unchanged: it is a disorder of movement and posture; it results from an abnormality in the brain; it is acquired early in life; and the condition is static at the time of recognition. The current definition and classification systems also recognize that the motor impairment is often accompanied by disturbances of sensation, perception, cognition, communication, behavior, epilepsy, and secondary musculoskeletal problems, all of which may significantly impact function. The diversity of clinical features enables CP to be described or classified in a variety of ways. However, challenges arise on adapting clinical classification for epidemiologic studies. For surveillances purposes, epidemiologists have developed systems aimed at improving reliability and enabling comparison of different populations. There are now several international surveillance networks that have collaborated in an effort to support international comparisons. Recent advances have been made toward incorporating measures of functioning into epidemiologic studies.

A variety of methods are used to ascertain cases and measure the prevalence of CP in the population. Surveillance systems in the United States, Europe, and Australia carry out ongoing, population-based record reviews using multiple community sources that diagnose, treat, or serve children with developmental disabilities. Systems in Europe and Australia also use other reporting methods. Incorporating information from multiple health, education, and service providers rather than relying on only one facility or one type of facility to identify children allows for more complete coverage of case identification in a defined population.

Identification of causal relationships in CP has been challenging. The causal pathways for CP are believed to be numerous and the etiology multifactorial. Risk factors are commonly categorized by the timing of their proposed occurrence: prenatal, perinatal, and postnatal. The leading prenatal and perinatal risk factors for CP are birth weight and gestational age. Other risk factors include neonatal encephalopathy, multiple pregnancy, infection and inflammation, and a variety of genetic factors. Population-based surveillance has enabled studies evaluating prevalence and risk factor relationships over time and within different risk subgroups. Population-based data on the longer-term consequences of CP are limited; it will be important in the future to use population-based methods to scrutinize the functional outcomes and consequences of CP in adults.

REFERENCES

1. Arneson C, Durkin M, Benedict R, et al. Brief report: prevalence of cerebral palsy - autism and developmental disabilities monitoring network, three sites. Disability and Health Journal 2009;2:45–8.
2. Charcot JM, Richer PMLP. Les deformes et les malades dans l'art. Paris: Lecrosnier et Babe; 1889.
3. Christensen E, Melchior J. Cerebral palsy – a clinical and neuropathological study. Clin Dev Med 1967;25:97–100.
4. Little WJ. Lectures on the deformity of the human frame. Lancet 1843;1:318–20.
5. Scherzer AL. In: Scherzer AL, editor. Early diagnosis and interventional therapy in cerebral palsy: an interdisciplinary age-focused approach. New York: Marcel Decker, Inc; 2001. p. 3–7, 9–10.

6. Little WJ. On the influence of abnormal parturition, difficult labor, premature birth and asphyxia neonatorum on the mental and physical condition of the child, especially in relation to deformities. Transactions of the Obstetrical Society of London 1862;3:293.

7. Osler W. The cerebral palsies of childhood. London: HK Lewis; 1889.

8. Freud S. Les diplegies cérébrales infantiles. Rev Neurol 1893;1:178–83.

9. Minear WL. A classification of cerebral palsy. Pediatrics 1956;18:841–52.

10. MacKeith RC, Polani PE. The Little Club: memorandum on terminology and classification of cerebral palsy. Cereb Palsy Bull 1959;5:27–35.

11. Bax MC. Terminology and classification of cerebral palsy. Dev Med Child Neurol 1964;11:295–7.

12. Evans P, Alberman E, Johnson A, et al. Standardization of recording and reporting cerebral palsy. Dev Med Child Neurol 1987;29:272.

13. Mutch L, Alberman E, Hagberg B, et al. Cerebral palsy epidemiology: where are we now and where are we going? [see comment]. Dev Med Child Neurol 1992;34:547–51.

14. Surveillance of Cerebral Palsy in Europe. a collaboration of cerebral palsy surveys and registers. Surveillance of Cerebral Palsy in Europe (SCPE) [see comment]. Dev Med Child Neurol 2000;42:816–24.

15. Rosenbaum P, Paneth N, Leviton A, et al. The definition and classification of cerebral palsy. Dev Med Child Neurol 2007;49(Suppl 109):8–14.

16. Blair E, Stanley F. The epidemiology of the cerebral palsies. In: Levene M, Chervenak F, editors. Fetal and neonatal neurology. 4th edition. Edinburgh: Churchill Livingstone Elsevier; 2009. p. 867–8.

17. Badawi N, Watson L, Petterson B, et al. What constitutes cerebral palsy? [see comment]. Dev Med Child Neurol 1998;40:520–7.

18. Howard J, Soo B, Graham HK, et al. Cerebral palsy in Victoria: motor types, topography and gross motor function. J Paediatr Child Health 2005;41:479–83.

19. Alberman E. Describing the cerebral palsies: methods of classifying and counting. In: Stanley F, Alberman E, editors. The epidemiology of the cerebral palsies. Philadelphia: JB Lippincott; 1984. p. 27–31.

20. Nelson K, Chang T. Is cerebral palsy preventable? Date of Publication: Apr 2008. Curr Opin Neurol 2008;21(2):129–35.

21. Shapiro BK. Cerebral palsy: a reconceptualization of the spectrum. J Pediatr 2004;145:S3–7.

22. Nelson KB, Ellenberg JH. Antecedents of cerebral palsy, I: univariate analysis of risks. Am J Dis Child 1985;139:1031–8.

23. Nelson KB, Ellenberg JH. Antecedents of cerebral palsy: multivariate analysis of risk. N Engl J Med 1986;315:81–6.

24. Plessis AJd, Volpe JJ. Perinatal brain injury in the preterm and term newborn. Curr Opin Neurol 2002;15:151–7.

25. Dammann O, Kuban KCK, Leviton A. Perinatal infection, fetal inflammatory response, white matter damage, and cognitive limitations in children born preterm. Ment Retard Dev Disabil Res Rev 2002;8:46–50.

26. Accardo PJ, Hoon AH Jr. The challenge of cerebral palsy classification: The ELGAN study. J Pediatr 2008;153(4):451–542.

27. Capute AJ, Shapiro BK, Palmer FB. Cerebral palsy: history and state of the art. In: Gottlieb M, Williams J, editors. Textbook of developmental pediatrics. New York: Plenum; 1987. p. 11–26.

28. World Health Organization. International classification of functioning, disability, and health (ICF), in. Geneva: World Health Organization; 2001.

29. Cans C, Dolk H, Platt MJ, et al. Recommendations from the SCPE collaborative group for defining and classifying cerebral palsy. Dev Med Child Neurol 2007;109:35–8.
30. Winter S, Autry A, Boyle C, et al. Trends in the prevalence of cerebral palsy in a population-based study. Pediatrics 2002;110:1220–5.
31. Yeargin-Allsopp M, Van Naarden Braun K, Doernberg NS, et al. Prevalence of cerebral palsy in 8-year-old children in three areas of the United States in 2002: a multisite collaboration. Pediatrics 2008;121:547–54.
32. Blair E, Badawi N, Watson L. Definition and classification of the cerebral palsies: the Australian view. Dev Med Child Neurol 2007;109:33–4.
33. Shevell MI, Majnemer A, Morin I. Etiologic yield of cerebral palsy: a contemporary case series. Pediatr Neurol 2003;28:352–9.
34. Cans C, De-la-Cruz J, Mermet M-A. Epidemiology of cerebral palsy. Paediatr Child Health 2008;18:393–8.
35. Gainsborough M, Surman G, Maestri G, et al. Validity and reliability of the guidelines of the surveillance of cerebral palsy in Europe for the classification of cerebral palsy. Dev Med Child Neurol 2008;50:828–31.
36. Bax M, Goldstein M, Rosenbaum P, et al. Proposed definition and classification of cerebral palsy, April 2005 [see comment]. Dev Med Child Neurol 2005;47:571–6.
37. Rosenbaum P, Paneth N, Leviton A, et al. A report: the definition and classification of cerebral palsy April 2006 [see comment] [erratum appears in Dev Med Child Neurol Suppl. 2007;49(6):480]. Dev Med Child Neurol 2007;109:8–14.
38. Palisano R, Rosenbaum P, Walter S, et al. Development and reliability of a system to classify gross motor function in children with cerebral palsy. Dev Med Child Neurol 1997;39:214–23.
39. Eliasson A, Krumlinde-Sundholm L, Rosblad B, et al. Manual Ability Classification System for children with cerebral palsy 4–18 years. Available at: http://www.macs.nu/. Accessed March 3, 2009.
40. Palisano R, Rosenbaum P, Bartlett DJ, et al. Gross Motor Function Classification System (GMFCS): expanded and revised, 2007. Available at: http://www.canchild.ca/Default.aspx?tabid=195. Accessed March 3, 2009.
41. Teutsh SM, Churchill RE. Principles and Practice of Public Health Surveillance. 2nd edition. Oxford: University Press; 2007.
42. The Cerebral Palsy Institute. Cerebral palsy register and surveillance survey report. Sydney, Australia: The Cerebral Palsy Institute; 2009.
43. Paneth N, Hong T, Korseniewski S. The descriptive epidemiology of cerebral palsy. Clin Perinatol 2006;33:251–67.
44. Murphy CC, Yeargin-Allsopp M, Decoufle P, et al. Prevalence of cerebral palsy among ten-year-old children in metropolitan Atlanta, 1985 through 1987. J Pediatr 1993;123:S13–20.
45. Yeargin-Allsopp M, Boyle CA, Van Naarden Braun K, et al. The epidemiology of developmental disabilities. In: Pasquale J, Accardo M, editors. Capute & Accardo's neurodevelopmental disabilities in infancy and childhood. 3rd edition, The spectrum of neurodevelopmental disabilities, Vol II. Baltimore: Paul H. Brookes Publishing Co; 2008. p. 76.
46. Bhasin TK, Brocksen S, Avchen RN, et al. Prevalence of four developmental disabilities among children aged 8 years–metropolitan Atlanta developmental disabilities surveillance program, 1996 and 2000 [erratum appears in MMWR Morb Mortal Wkly Rep. 2006 Feb 3;55(4):105-6]. MMWR Surveill Summ 2006;55:1–9.
47. Boyle CA, Yeargin-Allsopp M, Doernberg NS, et al. Prevalence of selected developmental disabilities in children 3–10 years of age: the Metropolitan Atlanta Developmental Disabilities Surveillance Program. MMWR Surveill Summ 1991;45(1):1–14.

48. Himmelmann K, Hagberg G, Beckung E, et al. The changing panorama of cerebral palsy in Sweden. IX. Prevalence and origin in the birth-year period 1995–1998. Acta Paediatr 2005;94:287–94.

49. American Academy of Pediatrics. Postnatal corticosteroids to treat or prevent chronic lung disease in preterm infants. Pediatrics 2002;109:330–8.

50. Wilson-Costello D, Friedman H, Minich N, et al. Improved neurodevelopmental outcomes for extremely low birth weight infants in 2000–2002 [see comment]. Pediatrics 2007;119:37–45.

51. Parkes J, Dolk H, Hill N, et al. Cerebral palsy in Northern Ireland: 1981–93. Paediatr Perinat Epidemiol 2001;15:278–86.

52. Topp M, Uldall P, Greisen G. Cerebral palsy births in eastern Denmark, 1987–90: implications for neonatal care. Paediatr Perinat Epidemiol 2001;15:271–7.

53. Surveillance of Cerebral Palsy in Europe. Prevalence and characteristics of children with cerebral palsy in Europe. Dev Med Child Neurol 2002;44:633–40.

54. Surveillance of Cerebral Palsy in Europe 1976-1990: Scientific Report. Grenoble: ISRN TIMC/RS-02-01-FR+SCPE; 2002.

55. Colver AF, Gibson M, Hey EN, et al. Increasing rates of cerebral palsy across the severity spectrum in north-east England 1964–1993. The North of England collaborative cerebral palsy survey. Arch Dis Child Fetal Neonatal Ed 2000;83:F7–12.

56. Robertson CMT, Watt M-J, Yasui Y. Changes in the prevalence of cerebral palsy for children born very prematurely within a population-based program over 30 years. JAMA 2007;297:2733–40.

57. Blair E, Watson L. Epidemiology of cerebral palsy. Semin Fetal Neonatal Med 2006;11:117–25.

58. Doyle LW, Anderson PJ. Victorian Infant Collaborative Study G: Improved neurosensory outcome at 8 years of age of extremely low birthweight children born in Victoria over three distinct eras. Arch Dis Child Fetal Neonatal Ed 2005;90:F484–8.

59. Drummond PM, Colver AF. Analysis by gestational age of cerebral palsy in singleton births in north-east England 1970–94. Paediatr Perinat Epidemiol 2002;16:172–80.

60. Vincer MJ, Allen AC, Joseph KS, et al. Increasing prevalence of cerebral palsy among very preterm infants: a population-based study. Pediatrics 2006;118:e1621–6.

61. Platt MJ, Cans C, Johnson A, et al. Trends in cerebral palsy among infants of very low birthweight (<1500 g) or born prematurely (<32 weeks) in 16 European centres: a database study [see comment]. Lancet 2007;369:43–50.

62. Nelson KB, Willoughby RE. Overview: infection during pregnancy and neurologic outcome in the child. Ment Retard Dev Disabil Res Rev 2002;8:1–2.

63. Hagberg B, Hagberg G, Beckung E, et al. Changing panorama of cerebral palsy in Sweden. VIII. Prevalence and origin in the birth year period 1991–94. Acta Paediatr 2001;90:271–7.

64. Hagberg B, Hagberg G. The changing panorama of cerebral palsy–bilateral spastic forms in particular. Acta Paediatr Suppl 1996;416:48–52.

65. Badawi N, Felix JF, Kurinczuk JJ, et al. Cerebral palsy following term newborn encephalopathy: a population-based study [see comment]. Dev Med Child Neurol 2005;47:293–8.

66. Bonellie SR, Currie D, Chalmers J. Comparison of risk factors for cerebral palsy in twins and singletons. Dev Med Child Neurol 2005;47:587–91.

67. Lidegaard O, Pinborg A, Andersen AN. Imprinting diseases and IVF: Danish National IVF cohort study. Humanit Rep 2005;20:950–4.

68. Pinborg A, Loft A, Schmidt L, et al. Neurological sequelae in twins born after assisted conception: controlled national cohort study [see comment]. BMJ 2004;329:311.

69. Hvidtjorn D, Grove J, Schendel DE, et al. Cerebral palsy among children born after in vitro fertilization: the role of preterm delivery–a population-based, cohort study. Pediatrics 2006;118:475–82.

70. Girard S, Kadhim H, Roy M, et al. Role of perinatal inflammation in cerebral palsy. Pediatr Neurol 2009;40(3):168–74.

71. Hagberg H, Mallard C, Jacobsson B. Role of cytokines in preterm labour and brain injury. BJOG 2005;112(Suppl 1):16–8.

72. Aaltonen R, Heikkinen T, Hakala K, et al. Transfer of proinflammatory cytokines across term placenta. Obstet Gynecol 2005;106:802–7.

73. Nelson KB, Dambrosia JM, Iovannisci DM, et al. Genetic polymorphisms and cerebral palsy in very preterm infants. Pediatr Res 2005;57:494–9.

74. Graham E, Holcroft C, Rai K, et al. Neonatal cerebral white matter injury in preterm infants is associated with culture positive infections and only rarely with metabolic acidosis. Am J Obstet Gynecol 2004;191:1305–10.

75. Kendall G, Peebles D. Acute fetal hypoia: the modulating effect of infection. Early Hum Dev 2005;81:27–34.

76. Stoll B, Hansen N, Adams-Chapman I, et al. Neurodevelopmental and growth impairment among extremely low-birth-weight infants with neonatal infection. JAMA 2004;292:2357–65.

77. Vohr B, Wright L, Poole W, et al. Neurodevelopmental outcomes of extremely low birth weight infants <23 weeks' gestation between 1993 and 1998. Pediatrics 2005;116:635–43.

78. Schaefer G. Genetics considerations in cerebral palsy. Semin Pediatr Neurol 2008;15(1):21–6.

79. Gibson CS, Maclennan AH, Dekker GA, et al. Candidate genes and cerebral palsy: a population-based study. Pediatrics 2008;122:1079–85.

80. Gibson CS, MacLennan AH, Goldwater PN, et al. The association between inherited cytokine polymorphisms and cerebral palsy. Am J Obstet Gynecol 2006;194:674.e1–11.

81. Nelson KB. Thrombophilias, perinatal stroke, and cerebral palsy. Clin Obstet Gynaecol 2006;49:875–84.

82. Nelson KB. Causative factors in cerebral palsy. Clin Obstet Gynecol 2008;51: 749–62.

83. Odding E, Roebroeck ME, Stam HJ. The epidemiology of cerebral palsy: incidence, impairments and risk factors. Disabil Rehabil 2006;28:183–91.

84. Fennell EB, Dikel TN. Cognitive and neuropsychological functioning in children with cerebral palsy. J Child Neurol 2001;16(1):58–63 [erratum appears in J Child Neurol 2001;16(3):225].

85. Wallace SJ. Epilepsy in cerebral palsy. Dev Med Child Neurol 2001;43:713–7.

86. Aram DM, Eisele JA. Limits to a left hemisphere explanation for specific language impairment. J Speech Hear Res 1994;37:824–30.

87. Ito J, Araki A, Tanaka H, et al. Intellectual status of children with cerebral palsy after elementary education. Pediatr Rehabil 1997;1:199–206.

88. Sigurdardottir S, Eiriksdottir A, Gunnarsdottir E, et al. Cognitive profile in young Icelandic children with cerebral palsy. Dev Med Child Neurol 2008;50:357–62.

89. Edebol-Tysk K. Epidemiology of spastic tetraplegic cerebral palsy in Sweden. I. Impairments and disabilities. Neuropediatrics 1989;20:41–5.

90. Vargha-Khadem F, Isaacs E, van der Werf S, et al. Development of intelligence and memory in children with hemiplegic cerebral palsy. The deleterious consequences of early seizures. Brain 1992;115(Pt 1):315–29.

91. Beckung E, Hagberg G, Uldall P, et al. Probability of walking in children with cerebral palsy in Europe. Pediatrics 2008;121:e187–92.

92. Parkes J, White-Koning M, Dickinson HO, et al. Psychological problems in children with cerebral palsy: a cross-sectional European study. J Child Psychol Psychiatry 2008;49:405–13.

93. Ashwal S, Russman BS, Blasco PA, et al. Practice parameter: diagnostic assessment of the child with cerebral palsy: report of the Quality Standards Subcommittee of the American Academy of Neurology and the Practice Committee of the Child Neurology Society [see comment]. Neurology 2004;62:851–63.

94. Hoon AH Jr. Neuroimaging in cerebral palsy: patterns of brain dysgenesis and injury. J Child Neurol 2005;20:936–9.

95. Nagae LM, Hoon AH Jr, Stashinko E, et al. Diffusion tensor imaging in children with periventricular leukomalacia: variability of injuries to white matter tracts. AJNR Am J Neuroradiol 2007;28:1213–22.

96. Yekutiel M, Jariwala M, Stretch P. Sensory deficit in the hands of children with cerebral palsy: a new look at assessment and prevalence. Dev Med Child Neurol 1994;36:619–24.

97. Cooper J, Majnemer A, Rosenblatt B, et al. The determination of sensory deficits in children with hemiplegic cerebral palsy. J Child Neurol 1995;10:300–9.

98. Wingert JR, Burton H, Sinclair RJ, et al. Tactile sensory abilities in cerebral palsy: deficits in roughness and object discrimination. Dev Med Child Neurol 2008;50:832–8.

99. Jahnsen R, Villien L, Aamodt G, et al. Musculoskeletal pain in adults with cerebral palsy compared with the general population. J Rehabil Med 2004;36:78–84.

100. McKearnan KA, Kieckhefer GM, Engel JM, et al. Pain in children with cerebral palsy: a review. J Neurosci Nurs 2004;36:252–9.

101. Russo RN, Miller MD, Haan E, et al. Pain characteristics and their association with quality of life and self-concept in children with hemiplegic cerebral palsy identified from a population register. Clin J Pain 2008;24:335–42.

102. Schenk-Rootlieb AJ, van Nieuwenhuizen O, van der Graaf Y, et al. The prevalence of cerebral visual disturbance in children with cerebral palsy. Dev Med Child Neurol 1992;34:473–80.

103. Pennefather PM, Tin W. Ocular abnormalities associated with cerebral palsy after preterm birth. Eye 2000;14:78–81.

104. Gisel E. Interventions and outcomes for children with dysphagia. Dev Disabil Res Rev 2008;14:165–73.

105. Reilly S, Skuse D, Poblete X. Prevalence of feeding problems and oral motor dysfunction in children with cerebral palsy: a community survey. J Pediatr 1996;129:877–82.

106. Venkateswaran S, Shevell MI. Comorbidities and clinical determinants of outcome in children with spastic quadriplegic cerebral palsy. Dev Med Child Neurol 2008;50:216–22.

107. Day SM, Strauss DJ, Vachon PJ, et al. Growth patterns in a population of children and adolescents with cerebral palsy [see comment]. Dev Med Child Neurol 2007;49:167–71.

108. Henderson RC, Kairalla JA, Barrington JW, et al. Longitudinal changes in bone density in children and adolescents with moderate to severe cerebral palsy. J Pediatr 2005;146:769–75.

109. Henderson RC, Gilbert SR, Clement ME, et al. Altered skeletal maturation in moderate to severe cerebral palsy [see comment]. Dev Med Child Neurol 2005;47:229–36.

110. Ozturk M, Oktem F, Kisioglu N, et al. Bladder and bowel control in children with cerebral palsy: case-control study. Croat Med J 2006;47:264–70.

111. Roijen LE, Postema K, Limbeek VJ, et al. Development of bladder control in children and adolescents with cerebral palsy [see comment]. Dev Med Child Neurol 2001;43:103–7.

112. Karaman MI, Kaya C, Caskurlu T, et al. Urodynamic findings in children with cerebral palsy. Int J Urol 2005;12:717–20.

113. Bross S, Honeck P, Kwon ST, et al. Correlation between motor function and lower urinary tract dysfunction in patients with infantile cerebral palsy. Neurourol Urodyn 2007;26:222–7.

114. Reid CJ, Borzyskowski M. Lower urinary tract dysfunction in cerebral palsy. Arch Dis Child 1993;68:739–42.

115. Van Naarden Braun K, Yeargin-Allsopp M, Lollar D. A multi-dimensional approach to the transition of children with developmental disabilities into young adulthood: the acquisition of adult social roles. Disabil Rehabil 2006;28:915–28.

116. Van Naarden Braun K, Yeargin-Allsopp M, Lollar D. Activity limitations among young adults with developmental disabilities: a population-based follow-up study. Res Dev Disabil 2009;30:179–91.

117. Wagner MM, Blackorby J. Transitioning from high school to work or college: how special education students fare. Future Child 1996;6(1):103–20.

118. Van Naarden Braun K, Doernberg N, Yeargin-Allsopp M. Co-occurrence of cerebral palsy and intellectual disabilities, hearing loss, vision impairment, and autism among children 8-years-old, metropolitan Atlanta developmental disabilities surveillance program, 2004 surveillance year. Dev Med Child Neurol 2009;51(Suppl 2):41.

119. Nordmark E, Hagglund G, Lagergren J. Cerebral palsy in southern Sweden I. Prevalence and clinical features. Acta Paediatr 2001;90:1271–6.

120. Sundrum R, Logan S, Wallace A, et al. Cerebral palsy and socioeconomic status: a retrospective cohort study [see comment]. Arch Dis Child 2005;90:15–8.

121. Serdaroglu A, Cansu A, Ozkan S, et al. Prevalence of cerebral palsy in Turkish children between the ages of 2 and 16 years. Dev Med Child Neurol 2006;48:413–6.

122. Watson L, Blaire E, Stanley F. Report of the Western Australia cerebral palsy register to birth year 1999 in Perth. In: TVW Telethon Institute for Child Health Research. Perth, Australia: 2009.

123. Andersen G, Irgens L, Haagaas I, et al. Cerebral palsy in Norway: prevalence, subtypes and severity. Eur J Paediatr Neurol 2008;12(1):4–13.

124. Himmelmann K, Beckung E, Hagberg G, et al. Gross and fine motor function and accompanying impairments in cerebral palsy. Dev Med Child Neurol 2006;48:417–23.

125. Beckung E, White-Koning M, Marcelli M, et al. Health status of children with cerebral palsy living in Europe: a multi-centre study. Child Care Health Dev 2008;34:806–14.

Common Medical Comorbidities Associated with Cerebral Palsy

David W. Pruitt, MD[a,b,*], Tobias Tsai, MD[a,b]

KEYWORDS

- Cerebral palsy • Seizures • Gastroesophageal reflux
- Sleep • Pain

The 2004 International Workshop of Definition and Classification of Cerebral Palsy definition includes the following: "The motor disorders of cerebral palsy are often accompanied by disturbances of sensation, perception, cognition, communication, and behaviors, by epilepsy, and by secondary musculoskeletal problems."[1] The Surveillance for Cerebral Palsy in Europe (SCPE) collaboration has reported that 31% of children with cerebral palsy (CP) have severe intellectual disability, 11% have severe visual disability, and 21% have epilepsy.[2] Thus, although CP is primarily a disorder of movement, many children with this diagnosis have other impairments that may affect their function, quality of life, and life expectancy. Children with a diagnosis of CP often have multiple medical issues that are best addressed by an interdisciplinary medical team, including a "medical home" with primary care physicians and additional assistance from multiple medical subspecialists. A comprehensive health plan implemented in the context of a well-defined "medical home" is a critical component to ensuring that the health needs of children with CP are adequately addressed.[3,4] Management of the multisystem-associated comorbidities requires a careful review of systems. Cerebral palsy is defined as a nonprogressive neurologic condition; however, as the child grows and matures physically and psychologically, the manifestations of the impairment are often not static. Recognition and appropriate

Disclosures: None.
[a] Division of Pediatric Rehabilitation, Department of Pediatrics, Cincinnati Children's Hospital Medical Center, University of Cincinnati College of Medicine, 3333 Burnet Avenue MLC 4009, Cincinnati, OH 45229-3039, USA
[b] Division of Pediatric Rehabilitation, Department of Physical Medicine & Rehabilitation, Cincinnati Children's Hospital Medical Center, University of Cincinnati College of Medicine, 3333 Burnet Avenue MLC 4009, Cincinnati, OH 45229-3039, USA
* Corresponding author. Division of Pediatric Rehabilitation, Department of Pediatrics, Cincinnati Children's Hospital Medical Center, University of Cincinnati College of Medicine, 3333 Burnet Avenue MLC 4003, Cincinnati, OH 45229-3039.
E-mail address: david.pruitt@cchmc.org (D.W. Pruitt).

Phys Med Rehabil Clin N Am 20 (2009) 453–467
doi:10.1016/j.pmr.2009.06.002
1047-9651/09/$ – see front matter © 2009 Elsevier Inc. All rights reserved.

management of these manifestations requires knowledge of the comorbidities accompanying CP. Management of the associated medical conditions that accompany CP can have a significant impact on the health, function, and quality of life of the child and family. A change in status of one medical condition may have significant impact on other signs and symptoms, for example, bladder infection or constipation may have effects on global spasticity. Coordination of care is required among the team members caring for a child with CP to optimize medical management, function, and quality of life. Identification of the more common medical issues that are addressed in a review of systems of a patient with CP is outlined below by general systems. Neuromuscular and musculoskeletal conditions are not addressed here as these areas are discussed within another article in this issue (see Damiano and colleagues).

NEUROLOGIC
Epilepsy

Epilepsy is common in individuals with CP. The prevalence reported in the literature varies depending on the type of seizure and on the type of CP, as well as on whether mental retardation is also present. Overall, the prevalence of seizures in children and adults with CP has been reported to be between 15% and 55%.[5–7] In individuals with CP and mental retardation, the prevalence rises to 71%.[8]

Epilepsy is particularly common in those with tetraplegic CP and in those with hemiplegic CP, with some studies finding epilepsy to be more prevalent in the former population,[5,8,9] and others finding it to be more prevalent in the latter.[7,10] In individuals with diplegic CP, prevalence has been estimated between 16% and 27%.[6,7] Age of onset tends to be earlier in those with spastic tetraplegia and diplegia, and later in those with hemiplegia.[7]

Given the variety of different lesions seen in different types of CP, it is not surprising that individuals with different types of CP might experience different types of seizures. Frequently these may secondarily generalize.[11] Partial epilepsy is the most common form of seizure activity in all children with CP, and is especially common in children with hemiplegia who have seizures[12] with a prevalence of around 70% in this specific population.[6] Generalized tonic-clonic seizures are more common in those individuals with spastic tetraplegia and diplegia.[7,8,11]

Electroencephalography (EEG) may assist in appropriate seizure diagnosis and optimal management of children with CP. In 1 study, abnormal EEG findings were assessed in 74 of 105 patients assessed with a diagnosis of CP, with slowing most often seen in children with tetraplegia and hemiplegia; most of the children with tetraplegia and diplegia demonstrate generalized abnormality.[7] In children who have definite seizures, traditional EEG may show epileptic spikes when there are nonepileptic involuntary movements related to the child's CP.[6] Video EEG may be useful to address this difficulty.

Interepileptiform discharges seen on EEG are also frequently observed in patients with CP, especially in those individuals with hemiplegia.[6] Although the appropriateness of "treating the EEG" is debated and data specific to individuals with CP are limited, interepileptiform discharges assessed during polysomnography have been found to be responsible for 23% of total sleep arousals in CP, and some investigators believe that such arousals may contribute to cognitive impairment.[13]

Overall management of epilepsy in individuals with CP, including pharmacologic management, is similar to that which would be undertaken in individuals without CP. One noteworthy consideration in this population, however, is the effect that baclofen, an often-used medication for spasticity management in individuals with CP, may have on seizures. Although it is an analog of g-aminobutyric acid type B (GABA-B), an inhibitory neurotransmitter, reports associate its use with an increase in seizures;[14] some indicate that this may be dose-related.[6] Evidence of the effectiveness of the ketogenic diet specifically in children with CP is lacking.

The prognosis for individuals with CP and epilepsy is variable. It is known that children with hemiplegic CP and epilepsy have lower full-scale intelligence quotient (IQ) scores than those with hemiplegic CP without epilepsy, as well as poorer performance on a variety of memory assessments.[15] Seizure relapse after antiepileptic drug discontinuation has been demonstrated to be significantly more likely in children with spastic hemiparesis than in individuals with spastic diplegia (61.5% versus 14.3%).[16] Evidence supports attempting discontinuation of antiepileptic drugs in children with CP after they have been seizure-free for at least 2 years.[16]

Visual Abnormalities

Children with CP have abnormalities of the visual sensory and motor pathways at rates exceeding those detected in neurologically normal children.[17] Studies have demonstrated that visual abnormalities in children with CP vary from 10% to 100%.[18,19] The premature infant may have severe visual impairment caused by retinopathy of prematurity (ROP). Children with less severe CP resemble the 1% to 4% of neurologically normal children in the general population who have infantile or refractive strabismus, whereas children with more severe CP have deficits that are either uncommon (eg, high myopia) or never seen (eg, dyskinetic strabismus) in neurologically normal children.[17] Worse visual acuity has been associated with increased levels of severity on the Gross Motor Function Classification System (GMFCS).[20,21] Children in GMFCS level V have been demonstrated to have a greater risk for high myopia, absence of any fusion, dyskinetic strabismus, more severe gaze dysfunction, optic neuropathy, and cerebral visual impairment.[17] Rates of optic neuropathy and gaze dysfunction also trend higher with higher GMFCS levels. Cerebral visual impairment, defined as bilateral, subnormal, best corrected visual acuity for age that could not be attributed to an ocular motor deficit (eg, nystagmus) or a structural defect of the anterior afferent visual pathway (eg, bilateral optic neuropathy), is present in up to 16% of children with CP, averaged across all GMFCS levels.[17]

All infants weighing less than 1500 g at birth or with a gestational age of 32 weeks or less should be screened for ROP by an ophthalmologist with experience in ROP screening until the blood vessels are mature, around 40 weeks from conception.[22] Children with CP should have yearly eye examinations, preferably by a pediatric ophthalmologist who is comfortable working with children with disabilities.[23]

Hearing Abnormalities

Hearing problems occur in approximately 30% to 40% of children with CP.[3,23] Hearing loss is known to be especially prevalent in children with CP with kernicterus, congenital infections, low birth weight, or severe hypoxic ischemic injury. Additional antecedents of hearing impairment in CP may also include prolonged artificial respiration after birth, persistent pulmonary hypertension, and the use of extracorporeal membrane oxygenation.[24,25] Conductive and sensori-neural impairments are found in children with CP, who should be screened by an audiologist.[26] Screening should generally be performed at intervals similar to those of all infants and children, but increased in those with risk factors such as congenital infections and treatment with ototoxic antibiotics.

Cognition

Given the heterogeneous nature of the causes and clinical manifestations of CP, it is difficult to generalize regarding the relationships between CP and cognitive function. Children with CP have been estimated to have associated mental retardation in the range from 30% to 50%.[27] Cognitive deficits tend to be most prevalent and severe in those with spastic tetraplegia, although children with spastic tetraplegia may have normal to near-normal intelligence. In children with spastic diplegia, there tends to be a general correlation between severity of motor deficit and level of cognitive deficit.[28] The presence of a seizure disorder may also be related to increased risk for cognitive deficits.[15,29] It is important to keep in mind that delayed or deficient language skills or dysarthria due to incoordination of muscles involved in speech or significant gross motor deficits can lead to false underestimation of intelligence.[30]

The use of standard measures of intelligence for assessing children with CP poses challenges, as the test results must be interpreted in the context of the motor, speech, visual, and auditory difficulties that may be present in these children. Difficulty with visual acuity and upper extremity motor impairment, for example, may impair hand-eye coordination and affect performance on several tests, and may contribute to a verbal-performance IQ split, with performance scores more affected due to decreased motor control. Children with spastic diplegia entering school, with IQ scores assessed before and 2 years after entering school, who were placed in regular classrooms, demonstrated an increase in verbal IQ, but not in performance IQ, in comparison to those children who were in special education classes. Children with CP in special education classrooms demonstrated higher mean increases in Wechsler performance IQs in comparison with those in regular classrooms. Thus, children with CP in regular classrooms revealed increasing disparity between verbal and performance IQs.[31] Advocacy for appropriate and optimal educational services at all levels of schooling and identification of potential resources to assist in obtaining these services should be provided, with anticipatory guidance given well before the start of kindergarten and through counseling at subsequent visits after the child is enrolled in school.

SLEEP

Sleep can be vulnerable due to many factors that are common in CP. Muscle spasms and other sources of musculoskeletal pain, decreased ability to change positions during the night, epilepsy and use of antiepileptic medications, and gastroesophageal reflux disease are a few of the many associated problems that can contribute to sleep disorders in children with CP. Abnormal sleep EEG patterns, including the absence of rapid eye movement (REM) sleep, abnormalities of the sleep spindles, and a high incidence of awakenings after sleep onset have been reported in 50% of children with CP.[32,33] Primary alterations in sleep architecture, possibly related to brainstem dysfunction, have also been reported in certain patients with athetoid CP.[34] Assessment of sleeping patterns and addressing associated factors that can contribute to difficulties is an important part of the review of systems in CP as there are many potential consequences of poor sleep including poor alertness and decreased cognitive performance. Children with CP may benefit from evaluation, after obtaining a thorough sleep history, including past medical history and risk factors, in a sleep disorders or pulmonary clinic setting. Polysomnography may be indicated, results of which may be helpful in guiding pharmacologic intervention.

PAIN

Pain is a common problem for individuals with CP, with more than half of adults and children with CP reporting pain as an ongoing health concern.[35] Children with CP experience more pain than the population norms and the presence of pain seems to persist into adulthood.[36] Children with more severe CP have been reported to have a higher pain frequency than children with less severe CP. Pain in children with CP has been associated with gender, occurring more commonly in girls, and with mobility, with accidental pain occurring more frequently in children with greater mobility. Adults with CP experience pain more frequently in the lower back, hips, and legs.[36,37] Pain in individuals with CP is often associated with educational and social consequences.[37] Despite these associations, there is a lack of information regarding pain characteristics in children with CP.[38]

Pain in children with CP can be difficult to assess, particularly in the nonverbal child. Possible sources of pain include a range from common causes, such as neuromuscular (muscle spasms), musculoskeletal (hip dislocation, scoliosis) and gastrointestinal (gastroesophageal reflux, constipation), to less common causes, such as dental (abscesses), ophthalmologic (corneal abrasions), and urologic (bladder spasms). Accurate assessment of pain in children with CP presents a challenge for health care providers, as it is difficult to obtain reliable measures of pain in many children because of cognitive immaturity, inability to separate pain from fear and anxiety, and the subjectivity of pain.[37] Numerous pain assessment scales have been developed that include self-report, physiologic measures, and behavioral measures and have been demonstrated to be appropriate across developmental levels. The overall validity of self-report of pain in children with CP is questionable, and observational assessment of pain is difficult because of idiosyncratic behaviors such as vocal abnormalities or facial peculiarities that can result in overestimates by those unfamiliar with an individual child's typical pattern of behavior.[37] Knowledge of behaviors and painful situations recognized by parents may help to better identify and subsequently manage pain in children with CP.[37–39] When these children present with pain, credible information can be obtained from a parent or guardian who knows the child well and these observations of behavior may be an acceptable alternative to self-report of pain.[40]

Often a thorough history and examination, with attention to the time course and temporal association (worse after meals or during diaper changes, for example) can suggest a potential cause and intervention.[35] This may lead to exploration of several empiric interventions before achieving comfort in the child, but families are often willing to participate in this process as long as they are involved and informed.

GASTROINTESTINAL

Gastrointestinal and nutritional problems are common in children with CP and can create considerable challenges for practitioners and caregivers. The ways in which those challenges are addressed can significantly impact the health and quality of life of the individual with CP, as well as the quality of life of the child's caregiver.

Motility Issues in Individuals with Cerebral Palsy

Because the enteric nervous system is rich, and the activity of enteric neurons is regulated by input from the central nervous system, motility abnormalities are frequently noted in individuals with CP.[41]

Esophageal dysmotility/gastroesophageal reflux/delayed gastric emptying

Gastroesophageal reflux disease (GERD), or the reflux of gastric contents into the esophagus, is a common problem in children with CP, with an estimated prevalence of up to 75%.[41,42] The reason for this high prevalence is likely multifactorial, primarily related to central nervous system impairment but also due to prolonged supine positioning in individuals with impaired mobility, and, for individuals receiving enteric tube feeds, the consistency of the diet being predominantly liquid. Both of these latter factors have been found to be contributors to GERD in normal infants, who have a similarly high prevalence.[43] Esophageal manometry has demonstrated alterations in esophageal motility in some children with CP, particularly those with spastic tetraplegia.[44]

Delayed gastric emptying has been reported in children with CP, with a prevalence of up to 67%.[45] Inadequately treated delayed gastric emptying has been hypothesized to interfere with the treatment of reflux, although some studies have found no relationship between gastroesophageal reflux and delayed gastric emptying.[41,46]

Vomiting and esophagitis are frequently noted symptoms of GERD in CP.[45] Tooth erosion due to the effects of reflux has been observed in children with CP, and, if not recognized and treated, may impair oral feeding.[47,48] GERD can also place the individual with CP at risk for chronic aspiration, especially when dysphagia is also present.

When GERD is present, conservative interventions to address positioning and the thickening of feeds, if appropriate and tolerated, may be appropriate first-line measures. In general, the same medications used for the treatment of reflux in neurologically unimpaired individuals, including proton pump inhibitors and histamine-2 receptor antagonists, are also appropriate for use in children with CP. Recent research supports a role for baclofen in the treatment of GERD. Baclofen, a GABA-B receptor agonist, inhibits triggering transient lower esophageal sphincter relaxation and also inhibits gastric emptying, reducing reflux.[49] Baclofen is also frequently used to treat spasticity, and may be especially useful in children with CP who have spasticity and GERD. If the symptoms of GERD are noted to persist despite medical therapies, surgical management is sometimes considered. Children with CP, compared with other individuals with neurologic impairment, have been demonstrated to be more likely to require surgical intervention for treatment of reflux.[50] Prophylactic fundoplication accompanying gastrostomy tube placement is occasionally advised because of concerns that gastrostomy, or the increase in feeding that often is enabled following gastrostomy, may worsen or precipitate GERD. However, a recent Cochrane review focusing on children with "neurologic impairment" generally and not specifically on those with a diagnosis of CP, indicated that robust scientific evidence is lacking as to whether fundoplication is beneficial in patients undergoing gastrostomy.[51] Other surgical procedures for the treatment of GERD, such as gastrojejunostomy tube placement or esophagogastric separation, are also occasionally used, but again there are little data specific to children with CP, as opposed to individuals with nonspecific "neurologic impairment."

Constipation

Constipation occurs in 26% to 90% of children with CP.[52,53] The cause of constipation in CP is multifactorial and may include immobility as well as slow colonic transit time.[52] Constipation is a significant problem in many children with CP and can contribute to other complaints, including pain, spasticity, feeding problems, irritability, poor appetite, and subsequent growth impairments. If not monitored and treated appropriately, ileus and permanent intestinal dysmotility can develop and, in extreme cases, can result in bowel perforation.[54] Inquiring about the bowel habits and bowel program, if one exists, is an important area of the review of systems in evaluating a child with CP. Historical information may reveal extensive time periods between bowel movements, frequent episodes of diarrhea, and characteristics of bowel movements as hard and pelletlike sometimes requiring digital disimpaction, all of which suggests that evaluation of the bowel program is necessary. Abdominal radiographs are sometimes helpful in assessing stool load, but often historical information will be effective in identifying bowel motility issues.

Treatment of bowel dysmotility also depends on information obtained during the clinical encounter. In cases of suspected obstipation, a clean-out program may be recommended, with use of medications impacting the upper and lower gastrointestinal tracts. The presence of hindgut dysmotility may lead some practitioners to limit or avoid the use of enemas associated with electrolyte derangements, such as tap water enemas and phosphate enemas; likewise, the presence of foregut dysmotility may lead some to avoid the administration of mineral oil by mouth due to aspiration risk. Typically, in cases of no significant concerns for either hindgut or foregut dysmotility, oral polyethylene glycol at doses of up to 1 mg/kg in addition to rectal suppository or enema is used. Pending good results following clean-out, a daily bowel program should be customized for the child. This program often includes a combination of stool softeners or oral promotility agents and a diet with the appropriate amounts of fiber and fluid. Attainment of regularly scheduled soft, formed bowel movements with minimal incontinence is the primary goal of the bowel program and timed evacuations are helpful in achieving this.

Feeding/Growth Issues

Feeding, and the challenges associated with it, is especially important in children with CP. Feeding dysfunction, as manifested by poor sucking, vomiting, and choking, may often precede the diagnosis of CP.[55] Problems with feeding may ultimately lead to problems with nutrition and subsequently to problems with growth.

Oropharyngeal dysphagia

The ability to form and manipulate a bolus and then to swallow it safely is a complex task that involves the coordination of multiple muscles that receive input from the cranial nerves (V, VII, and IX-XII). Severity of motor impairment, in general, is associated with dysphagia. Children classified at GMFCS level V (most severe) have been demonstrated to have more significant dysphagia than those at GMFCS level IV.[56] An impairment in the ability to swallow often places the child at risk for aspiration, frequently leading to respiratory infection. Although esophageal reflux may also contribute to aspiration, direct aspiration as a result of oropharyngeal dysfunction is more strongly associated with respiratory infection than esophageal reflux.[57] Up to 97% of nonambulatory children with CP and dysphagia have been demonstrated to be silent aspirators.[58]

The need for accurate assessment of the risk of aspiration is a critical reason for a proper evaluation of swallowing. In general, evaluation of dysphagia in the child with CP is similar to that for other children with dysphagia. Because children with CP often have abnormal tone, attention to positioning is particularly important when trying to optimize oral feedings.

Other difficulties with self-feeding may occur because motor impairments can make such feeding difficult or even impossible. Children with oropharyngeal dysphagia may eat more slowly and this may lead to longer mealtimes.[59,60] In children with severe spastic tetraplegia, feeding can be the most time-consuming basic care need.[61]

Children with dysphagia may prefer or be prescribed softer food textures and it is important to consider that softer foods may be less calorically dense, further contributing to inadequate caloric intake.

Enteric tube feeding

In children with CP in whom swallowing is not safe enough to allow oral feeding due to risk of aspiration, or in whom difficulties with feeding make it impossible or impractical to take in adequate calories by mouth, enteric tube feeds may be considered. This decision is often difficult, for the parent of the child for whom the procedure is being considered and for the practitioner caring for the child, because there are currently no randomized controlled trials addressing this issue.[41,62,63] A recent longitudinal, prospective, multicenter cohort study, although not randomized or blinded, found statistically significant and clinically important increases in weight gain and subcutaneous fat deposition and reported that almost all parents noted a significant improvement in their child's health after gastrostomy tube placement and a significant reduction in time spent feeding.[64] Although promising, further studies are needed to gain a better understanding of optimal feeding management for children with CP.

Growth and nutrition in children with cerebral palsy

With the knowledge that increased caloric intake will likely be helpful in improving growth, the practitioner is still faced with the question of what is considered "appropriate" growth for the child with CP. This question may be more obvious in the case of the child with severe spastic tetraplegia, but in fact it is an important question across the spectrum of children with CP, with poor growth observed at all levels of severity. Children with mild CP are at risk, with undernourishment demonstrated in up to 30% of children with hemiplegia or diplegia.[65] The analysis is further complicated as any assessment of appropriate caloric intake for growth needs to take into account that children with CP do not necessarily have the same caloric requirements as their peers in the general population. A high degree of variability in total energy expenditure (TEE) has been demonstrated in adults with CP, which appears largely attributable to high interindividual variation in energy expended in physical activity, thus making it difficult to provide general guidelines for energy requirements for this population.[66] Ambulation status has been shown to be an important predictor of TEE and should be taken into account when estimating energy requirements.[66] Formulas for calculating energy expenditure that take into account factors such as muscle tone, activity, and ambulation have been developed for adolescents with CP.[67] In assessing linear growth in children with CP, one must take into account that height or length may be difficult to obtain reliably due to the presence of contractures; formulas using segmental measures have been developed.[68] Body mass index (BMI; calculated as the weight in kilograms divided by height in meters squared) may not be a good indicator of nutrition in children with CP, primarily due to decreased muscle mass and decreased bone density.[69] Because of these considerations, it may not be appropriate to use standard growth charts based on a nonneurologically impaired population. Growth charts for children with CP have been created, with some published in a usable form for clinicians.[70,71]

Other indicators of nutrition frequently used in the general population, but found to be unreliable in children with CP, include serum prealbumin and albumin concentrations. There is little to no correlation of these values with anthropometric measures (eg, skinfolds, midarm fat area), growth (height), severity of CP, feeding dysfunction, or general health.[72] Several measures of nutritional status, including weight-for-height percentiles, arm circumference, BMI, lean BMI, head circumference to arm circumference ratio, triceps and subscapular skinfold thickness, have been evaluated and triceps skinfold thickness less than 10% for age/sex has been identified as the best indicator of malnutrition in children with CP.[73]

Micronutrient deficiencies in children with CP have been identified and associated with a low intake of iron, folate, niacin, calcium, vitamin E, and vitamin D, even among those who were receiving nutritional supplements.[74] Similarly, decreased levels of vitamin D and calcium in nonambulatory tube-fed children with CP have been identified.[75] (A detailed discussion of vitamin D and calcium and their relationship to bone growth in children with CP is provided in Houlihan and colleagues, this issue.)

Although most studies on malnutrition in children with CP focus on the problems associated with being underweight, some children with CP may be overweight. There is a rising prevalence of obesity (7.7%–16.5% during the past decade, and comparable to the general population during the same time period) in ambulatory children with CP.[76] This is especially significant as heavier children with CP may be less well equipped to handle the impact of increased weight, as indicated by a decrease in gait speed and an increase in VO_2.[77]

Growth in children with CP is unquestionably a complex issue, and currently there are few data to guide clinicians regarding what constitutes ideal, or even adequate, growth and nutritional status in this population.[69] However complex, it is an issue worth tackling, because data suggest that improved growth correlates with improvements in gross motor function measure (GMFM) scores and in measures of social participation.[78,79]

Sialorrhea

Sialorrhea, or drooling, is a problem for many children with CP, particularly in those with spastic tetraplegia. Reasons for drooling can include low oral muscle tone with poor lip closure, inadequate jaw closure, postural problems, dysphagia, inability to recognize salivary spill, and dental malocclusion. Effects of drooling can include chapping of the skin around the mouth, dehydration, dental enamel erosion, and odor, as well as social stigmatization, which can be significant for the family and the child.[80] A spectrum of treatment options is available for reduction of drooling. Conservative management including oral motor therapy with occupational or speech therapy is often the first line of treatment. Anticholinergic medication, such as glycopyrrolate or scopolamine patches, blocks parasympathetic innervation to the salivary glands and can be used. Side effects of these medications, including blurred vision, urinary retention, and sedation with glycopyrrolate, and heat insensitivity and increased irritability with scopolamine, often result in discontinuation. Focal treatment with botulinum toxin injections into the parotid and submandibular glands is another treatment option that is becoming more used, however it is limited due to the duration of its effectiveness. Surgical interventions including salivary gland excision, salivary duct ligation and duct rerouting are additional options, with limitations including discomfort and accelerated tooth decay.[81]

Dental

Dental problems in children with CP include pain, enamel erosion, and malocclusion, as above. Children with CP are additionally at increased risk for dental problems due to abnormal oral motor reflexes, swallowing difficulties that lead to retention of food particles in the mouth, and medications with detrimental influences on the oral environment. Regular dental care should be provided every 6 months. Positioning challenges can often be met without use of a general anesthetic. However, for some children with CP, anesthesia is required to provide complete evaluation and restorative care, with the major goal of preventing problems associated with poor dental health, including pain, decreased appetite and poor nutrition, and infection.[82]

RESPIRATORY

Children with CP have an increased incidence of primary respiratory disorders due to the nature of neurologic and anatomic dysfunction that is present in varying degrees. Chronic pulmonary complications can include recurrent pneumonia, atelectasis, bronchiectasis, and restrictive lung disease. One of the most common pulmonary symptoms is noisy breathing, which can be associated with anatomic or functional obstructions, excessive secretions secondary to gastroesophageal reflux or swallowing dysfunction, ineffective cough, or a combination of 2 or more of these factors. Airway hyposensitivity and ineffective cough can contribute to ineffective clearance of secretions from the respiratory tract and subsequent wheezing, pneumonia, and atelectasis. Chronic accumulation of secretions can lead to bronchiectasis, a condition of permanently dilated and damaged airways.[83]

A complete pulmonary assessment should include a thorough history including information related to respiratory events encountered from birth, including the presence of meconium aspiration, hyaline membrane disease, supplemental oxygen need, bronchopulmonary dysplasia, tracheomalacia, laryngomalacia, and time of any ventilator support. Inquiries regarding childhood pulmonary issues should include the presence or absence of recurrent lower respiratory tract infections, atopy, wheezing, sleeping disturbances, gastroesophageal reflux with aspiration, upper respiratory infections related to recurrent ear or sinus infections, or exposure to potential environmental irritants to the lung.[83]

ENDOCRINE

Puberty occurs in most adolescents with CP within the normal age range. Adolescents with CP with cognitive deficits may require assistance in understanding pubertal changes as well as the strong emotions that accompany these changes.[23] The American Academy of Pediatrics consensus is that sexuality should be discussed with children with disabilities to protect them from exploitation, sexually transmitted diseases, and unplanned pregnancies.[84] Objectives of the consensus statement on sexuality education include teaching children and adolescents with disabilities how to express physical affection in a manner appropriate to their chronologic, rather than developmental, age; discouraging hugging strangers; teaching what is appropriate touch from others; and when to alert parents that the inappropriate touch is occurring.[84]

UROLOGY

Children with CP are at risk for several problems related to the urinary tract, including incontinence, urgency, frequency, difficulty with initiating void, retention, and infections.[54] Spasticity and hyperreflexia of the skeletal muscles may be accompanied by spasticity of the detrusor, leading to small, frequent voids and a contracted, low-capacity bladder. More than one third of children with CP present with dysfunctional voiding symptoms.[85] The predominant urodynamic abnormality is classified as a pure upper motor neuron lesion with neurogenic detrusor activity, followed by detrusor sphincter dyssynergia.[86] Recognizing problems with lower urinary tract function and preventing damage to the upper urinary tract are important areas of management in the care of children with CP. The likelihood of discovering a urinary tract abnormality in children with CP who do not have symptoms of a urinary disorder is small, and therefore routine screening tests or routine referral of asymptomatic children with CP to a urologist is not recommended.[87]

Primary incontinence has been reported in 23.5% of children and adolescents with CP between the ages of 4 and 18 years.[32] The attainment of continence involves maturation of the urinary tract and the autonomic nervous system, as well as of cortical functions. Intellectual, communication, and fine motor skills are also required for children with CP to access the bathroom and manage undressing. Accommodations such as adaptive equipment including commodes, raised toilet seats, handrails, and clothing modifications also assist in achieving and maintaining continence.

SUMMARY

The medical issues associated with the diagnosis of CP can have significant interplay with the neuromuscular issues that most physiatrists manage in the clinical setting. Identification and appropriate management of these common comorbidities is helpful in the treatment from the primary care and subspecialist viewpoints and can have significant impact on the quality of life of the patient and family. Some of these issues are prevalent across all GMFCS levels of severity, whereas others are focused more on those with classifications of GMFCS IV and V. Performance of a complete review of systems to address the potentially complex medical comorbidities and subsequent application of appropriate screening tools can assist in achieving optimal outcomes for children with CP and their families.

REFERENCES

1. Rosenbaum P, Paneth N, Leviton A, et al. A report: the definition and classification of cerebral palsy April 2006. Dev Med Child Neurol Suppl 2007;109:8–14.
2. Cans C. Surveillance of cerebral palsy in Europe: a collaboration of cerebral palsy surveys and registers. Dev Med Child Neurol 2000;42:816–24.
3. Pellegrino L. Cerebral palsy. In: Batshaw ML, Pellegrino L, Roizen NJ, editors. Children with disabilities. 6th edition. Baltimore (MD): Paul H. Brookes Publishing Co.; 2007. p. 387–408.
4. Cooley WC. Providing a primary care medical home for children and youth with cerebral palsy. Pediatrics 2004;114(4):1106–13.
5. Odding E, Roebroeck ME, Stam HJ. The epidemiology of cerebral palsy: incidence, impairments and risk factors. Disabil Rehabil 2006;28(4):183–91.
6. Wallace SJ. Epilepsy in cerebral palsy. Dev Med Child Neurol 2001;43(10):713–7.
7. Singhi P, Jagirdar S, Khandelwal N, et al. Epilepsy in children with cerebral palsy. J Child Neurol 2003;18(3):174–9.
8. Hadjipanayis A, Hadjichristodoulou C, Youroukos S. Epilepsy in patients with cerebral palsy. Dev Med Child Neurol 1997;39(10):659–63.
9. Kwong KL, Wong SN, So KT. Epilepsy in children with cerebral palsy. Pediatr Neurol 1998;19(1):31–6.
10. Bruck I, Antoniuk SA, Spessatto A, et al. Epilepsy in children with cerebral palsy. Arq Neuropsiquiatr 2001;59(1):35–9.
11. Kulak W, Sobaniec W. Risk factors and prognosis of epilepsy in children with cerebral palsy in north-eastern Poland. Brain Dev 2003;25(7):499–506.
12. Carlsson M, Hagberg G, Olsson I. Clinical and aetiological aspects of epilepsy in children with cerebral palsy. Dev Med Child Neurol 2003;45(6):371–6.
13. Jaseja H. Cerebral palsy: interictal epileptiform discharges and cognitive impairment. Clin Neurol Neurosurg 2007;109(7):549–52.

14. Hansel DE, Hansel CR, Shindle MK, et al. Oral baclofen in cerebral palsy: possible seizure potentiation? Pediatr Neurol 2003;29(3):203–6.
15. Vargha-Khadem F, Isaacs E, van der Werf S, et al. Development of intelligence and memory in children with hemiplegic cerebral palsy. The deleterious consequences of early seizures. Brain 1992;115(Pt 1):315–29.
16. Delgado MR, Riela AR, Mills J, et al. Discontinuation of antiepileptic drug treatment after two seizure-free years in children with cerebral palsy. Pediatrics 1996;97(2):192–7.
17. Ghasia F, Brunstrom J, Gordon M, et al. Frequency and severity of visual sensory and motor deficits in children with cerebral palsy: gross motor function classification scale. Invest Ophthalmol Vis Sci 2008;49(2):572–80.
18. Guzzetta A, Mercuri E, Cioni G. Visual disorders in children with brain lesions: 2. Visual impairment associated with cerebral palsy. Eur J Paediatr Neurol 2001; 5(3):115–9.
19. Stiers P, Vanderkelen R, Vanneste G, et al. Visual-perceptual impairment in a random sample of children with cerebral palsy. Dev Med Child Neurol 2002; 44(6):370–82.
20. Himmelmann K, Beckung E, Hagberg G, et al. Gross and fine motor function and accompanying impairments in cerebral palsy. Dev Med Child Neurol 2006;48(6): 417–23.
21. Nordmark E, Hagglund G, Lagergren J. Cerebral palsy in southern Sweden II. Gross motor function and disabilities. Acta Paediatr 2001;90(11):1277–82.
22. American Academy of Pediatrics, American Academy of Ophthalmology, American Association for Pediatric Ophthalmology and Strabismus. Policy statement: screening examination of the premature infants for retinopathy of prematurity. Pediatrics 2006;117:572–6.
23. Jones MW, Morgan E, Shelton JE. Primary care of the child with cerebral palsy: a review of systems (part II). J Pediatr Health Care 2007;21(4):226–37.
24. Graziani LJ, Baumgart S, Desai S, et al. Clinical antecedents of neurologic and audiologic abnormalities in survivors of neonatal extracorporeal membrane oxygenation. J Child Neurol 1997;12(7):415–22.
25. Borg E. Perinatal asphyxia, hypoxia, ischemia and hearing loss. An overview. Scand Audiol 1997;26(2):77–91.
26. Green L, Greenberg G, Hurwitz E. Primary care of children with cerebral palsy. Clin Fam Pract 2003;5(2):467–91.
27. Green LB, Hurvitz EA. Cerebral palsy. Phys Med Rehabil Clin N Am 2007;18(4): 859–82, vii.
28. Menkes JH, Sarnat HB. Perinatal asphyxia and trauma. In: Menkes JH, Samat HB, editors. Child neurology. Philadephia: Lippincott Williams & Wilkins; 2000. p. 401–66.
29. Zafeiriou DI, Kontopoulos EE, Tsikoulas I. Characteristics and prognosis of epilepsy in children with cerebral palsy. J Child Neurol 1999;14(5):289–94.
30. Fennell EB, Dikel TN. Cognitive and neuropsychological functioning in children with cerebral palsy. J Child Neurol 2001;16(1):58–63.
31. Ito J, Araki A, Tanaka H, et al. Intellectual status of children with cerebral palsy after elementary education. Pediatr Rehabil 1997;1(4):199–206.
32. Murphy N, Such-Neibar T. Cerebral palsy diagnosis and management: the state of the art. Curr Probl Pediatr Adolesc Health Care 2003;33(5):146–69.
33. Newman CJ, O'Regan M, Hensey O. Sleep disorders in children with cerebral palsy. Dev Med Child Neurol 2006;48(7):564–8.

34. Hayashi M, Inoue Y, Iwakawa Y, et al. REM sleep abnormalities in severe athetoid cerebral palsy. Brain Dev 1990;12(5):494–7.
35. Dodge NN. Cerebral palsy: medical aspects. Pediatr Clin North Am 2008;55(5): 1189–207, ix.
36. Russo RN, Miller MD, Haan E, et al. Pain characteristics and their association with quality of life and self-concept in children with hemiplegic cerebral palsy identified from a population register. Clin J Pain 2008;24(4):335–42.
37. Houlihan CM, O'Donnell M, Conaway M, et al. Bodily pain and health-related quality of life in children with cerebral palsy. Dev Med Child Neurol 2004;46(5):305–10.
38. Tervo RC, Symons F, Stout J, et al. Parental report of pain and associated limitations in ambulatory children with cerebral palsy. Arch Phys Med Rehabil 2006; 87(7):928–34.
39. Hadden KL, von Baeyer CL. Pain in children with cerebral palsy: common triggers and expressive behaviors. Pain 2002;99(1–2):281–8.
40. American Academy of Pediatrics, Committee on Psychosocial Aspects of Child and Family Health; American Pain Society Task Force on Pain in Infants, Children, and Adolescents. The assessment and management of acute pain in infants, children, and adolescents. Pediatrics 2001;108(3):793–7.
41. Sullivan PB. Gastrointestinal disorders in children with neurodevelopmental disabilities. Dev Disabil Res Rev 2008;14(2):128–36.
42. Ceriati E, De Peppo F, Ciprandi G, et al. Surgery in disabled children: general gastroenterological aspects. Acta Paediatr Suppl 2006;95(452):34–7.
43. Kirby M, Noel RJ. Nutrition and gastrointestinal tract assessment and management of children with dysphagia. Semin Speech Lang 2007;28(3):180–9.
44. Gustafsson PM, Tibbling L. Gastro-oesophageal reflux and oesophageal dysfunction in children and adolescents with brain damage. Acta Paediatr 1994;83(10):1081–5.
45. Del Giudice E, Staiano A, Capano G, et al. Gastrointestinal manifestations in children with cerebral palsy. Brain Dev 1999;21(5):307–11.
46. Spiroglou K, Xinias I, Karatzas N, et al. Gastric emptying in children with cerebral palsy and gastroesophageal reflux. Pediatr Neurol 2004;31(3):177–82.
47. Shaw L, Weatherill S, Smith A. Tooth wear in children: an investigation of etiological factors in children with cerebral palsy and gastroesophageal reflux. ASDC J Dent Child 1998;65(6):484–6, 439.
48. Su JM, Tsamtsouris A, Laskou M. Gastroesophageal reflux in children with cerebral palsy and its relationship to erosion of primary and permanent teeth. J Mass Dent Soc 2003;52(2):20–4.
49. Omari TI, Benninga MA, Sansom L, et al. Effect of baclofen on esophagogastric motility and gastroesophageal reflux in children with gastroesophageal reflux disease: a randomized controlled trial. J Pediatr 2006;149(4):468–74.
50. Novotny NM, Jester AL, Ladd AP. Preoperative prediction of need for fundoplication before gastrostomy tube placement in children. J Pediatr Surg 2009;44(1): 173–6 [discussion: 176–7].
51. Vernon-Roberts A, Sullivan PB. Fundoplication versus post-operative medication for gastro-oesophageal reflux in children with neurological impairment undergoing gastrostomy. Cochrane Database Syst Rev 2007;(1):CD006151.
52. Park ES, Park CI, Cho SR, et al. Colonic transit time and constipation in children with spastic cerebral palsy. Arch Phys Med Rehabil 2004;85(3):453–6.
53. Agnarsson U, Warde C, McCarthy G, et al. Anorectal function of children with neurological problems. II: cerebral palsy. Dev Med Child Neurol 1993;35(10):903–8.

54. Pellegrino L. Well-child care and health maintenance. In: Dormans JP, Pellegrino L, editors. Caring for children with cerebral palsy. Baltimore: Paul H. Brookes Publishing Co.; 1998. p. 71–93.

55. Reilly S, Skuse D. Characteristics and management of feeding problems of young children with cerebral palsy. Dev Med Child Neurol 1992;34(5):379–88.

56. Calis EA, Veugelers R, Sheppard JJ, et al. Dysphagia in children with severe generalized cerebral palsy and intellectual disability. Dev Med Child Neurol 2008;50(8):625–30.

57. Morton RE, Wheatley R, Minford J. Respiratory tract infections due to direct and reflux aspiration in children with severe neurodisability. Dev Med Child Neurol 1999;41(5):329–34.

58. Rogers B, Arvedson J, Buck G, et al. Characteristics of dysphagia in children with cerebral palsy. Dysphagia 1994;9(1):69–73.

59. Wright RE, Wright FR, Carson CA. Videofluoroscopic assessment in children with severe cerebral palsy presenting with dysphagia. Pediatr Radiol 1996;26(10):720–2.

60. Gisel E. Interventions and outcomes for children with dysphagia. Dev Disabil Res Rev 2008;14(2):165–73.

61. Edebol-Tysk K. Evaluation of care-load for individuals with spastic tetraplegia. Dev Med Child Neurol 1989;31(6):737–45.

62. Sullivan PB. Gastrostomy and the disabled child. Dev Med Child Neurol 1992; 34(6):552–5.

63. Sleigh G, Sullivan PB, Thomas AG. Gastrostomy feeding versus oral feeding alone for children with cerebral palsy. Cochrane Database Syst Rev 2004;(2):CD003943.

64. Sullivan PB, Juszczak E, Bachlet AM, et al. Gastrostomy tube feeding in children with cerebral palsy: a prospective, longitudinal study. Dev Med Child Neurol 2005;47(2):77–85.

65. Stallings VA, Charney EB, Davies JC, et al. Nutritional status and growth of children with diplegic or hemiplegic cerebral palsy. Dev Med Child Neurol 1993; 35(11):997–1006.

66. Johnson RK, Hildreth HG, Contompasis SH, et al. Total energy expenditure in adults with cerebral palsy as assessed by doubly labeled water. J Am Diet Assoc 1997;97(9):966–70.

67. Bandini LG, Schoeller DA, Fukagawa NK, et al. Body composition and energy expenditure in adolescents with cerebral palsy or myelodysplasia. Pediatr Res 1991;29(1):70–7.

68. Stevenson RD. Use of segmental measures to estimate stature in children with cerebral palsy. Arch Pediatr Adolesc Med 1995;149(6):658–62.

69. Kuperminc MN, Stevenson RD. Growth and nutrition disorders in children with cerebral palsy. Dev Disabil Res Rev 2008;14(2):137–46.

70. Day SM, Strauss DJ, Vachon PJ, et al. Growth patterns in a population of children and adolescents with cerebral palsy. Dev Med Child Neurol 2007;49(3):167–71.

71. Stevenson RD, Conaway M, Chumlea WC, et al. Growth and health in children with moderate-to-severe cerebral palsy. Pediatrics 2006;118(3):1010–8.

72. Lark RK, Williams CL, Stadler D, et al. Serum prealbumin and albumin concentrations do not reflect nutritional state in children with cerebral palsy. J Pediatr 2005; 147(5):695–7.

73. Samson-Fang LJ, Stevenson RD. Identification of malnutrition in children with cerebral palsy: poor performance of weight-for-height centiles. Dev Med Child Neurol 2000;42(3):162–8.

74. Hillesund E, Skranes J, Trygg KU, et al. Micronutrient status in children with cerebral palsy. Acta Paediatr 2007;96(8):1195–8.

75. Duncan B, Barton LL, Lloyd J, et al. Dietary considerations in osteopenia in tube-fed nonambulatory children with cerebral palsy. Clin Pediatr (Phila) 1999;38(3): 133–7.
76. Rogozinski BM, Davids JR, Davis RB, et al. Prevalence of obesity in ambulatory children with cerebral palsy. J Bone Joint Surg Am 2007;89(11):2421–6.
77. Plasschaert F, Jones K, Forward M. The effect of simulating weight gain on the energy cost of walking in unimpaired children and children with cerebral palsy. Arch Phys Med Rehabil 2008;89(12):2302–8.
78. Campanozzi A, Capano G, Miele E, et al. Impact of malnutrition on gastrointestinal disorders and gross motor abilities in children with cerebral palsy. Brain Dev 2007;29(1):25–9.
79. Samson-Fang L, Fung E, Stallings VA, et al. Relationship of nutritional status to health and societal participation in children with cerebral palsy. J Pediatr 2002; 141(5):637–43.
80. Hockstein NG, Samadi DS, Gendron K, et al. Sialorrhea: a management challenge. Am Fam Physician 2004;69(11):2628–34.
81. Toder DS. Respiratory problems in the adolescent with developmental delay. Adolesc Med 2000;11(3):617–31.
82. Greenhill W. Dental care for children with disabilities. In: Rudolph CD, Rudolph AM, Hostetter MK, et al, editors. Rudolph's pediatrics. New York: McGraw-Hill; 2003. p. 541–2.
83. Sobus KM, Horan SM, Warren RH. Respiratory management of neuromuscular diseases. In: Alexander MA, Molnar GE, editors, Physical medicine and rehabilitation: state of the art reviews, Vol. 14. Philadelphia: Hanley & Belfus; 2000. p. 285–300.
84. American Academy of Pediatrics. Sexuality education of children and adolescents with developmental disabilities. Pediatrics 1996;97:275–8.
85. Karaman MI, Kaya C, Caskurlu T, et al. Urodynamic findings in children with cerebral palsy. Int J Urol 2005;12(8):717–20.
86. Decter RM, Bauer SB, Khoshbin S, et al. Urodynamic assessment of children with cerebral palsy. J Urol 1987;138(4 Pt 2):1110–2.
87. Brodak PP, Scherz HC, Packer MG, et al. Is urinary tract screening necessary for patients with cerebral palsy? J Urol 1994;152(5 Pt 1):1586–7.

New Clinical and Research Trends in Lower Extremity Management for Ambulatory Children with Cerebral Palsy

Diane L. Damiano, PhD, PT[a],*, Katharine E. Alter, MD[a,b],
Henry Chambers, MD[c]

KEYWORDS

- Physical therapy • Medication • Botulinum toxin • Gait
- Orthopedic surgery • Training • Spasticity

OVERVIEW OF CURRENT CARE OF MOTOR DISORDERS IN CEREBRAL PALSY

Cerebral palsy (CP) is the most prevalent physical disability originating in childhood. The latest figures in the United States indicate that the incidence of CP is 3.6 per 1000 children, with males affected to a greater extent than females.[1] Because no cure is yet available or imminent for CP, the motor disability persists throughout the lifespan and interferes with normal developmental and aging processes, which alter its presentation with time. The current standard of care for the motor disorder in CP consists of regular physical therapy, followed by multiple, and often concurrent, medical and surgical interventions, most intensively in early childhood through preadolescence. Although a growing list of treatments have been shown to individually improve motor outcomes, few definitive practice guidelines have been proposed for the management of CP due to limited and fragmented scientific evidence to support multidisciplinary (combined) intervention approaches. Consequently, tremendous variation exists among different practitioners, settings, and geographical areas in

[a] Functional & Applied Biomechanics Section, Clinical Center, National Institutes of Health, 10 Center Drive, Room 1-1469, Bethesda, MD 20892, USA
[b] Rehabilitation Medicine Department, National Institute for Child Health and Human Development, National Institutes of Health, Bethesda, MD 20892, USA
[c] Department of Orthopedic Surgery, University of California at San Diego, Rady Children's Hospital, 3030 Children's Way, San Diego, CA 92123, USA
* Corresponding author. Functional & Applied Biomechanics Section, Clinical Center, National Institutes of Health, 10 Center Drive, Room 1-1469, Bethesda, MD 20892, USA.
E-mail address: damianod@cc.nih.gov (D.L. Damiano).

Phys Med Rehabil Clin N Am 20 (2009) 469–491
doi:10.1016/j.pmr.2009.04.005
1047-9651/09/$ – see front matter © 2009 Elsevier Inc. All rights reserved.

the types of treatments prescribed, the timing and sequencing of interventions, and the range of treatment intensity or frequency. Choice of, and response to, intervention is further complicated by the fact that CP is not a single disease entity with a known causal pathway; it is, instead, a heterogeneous group of disorders with varying etiologies, brain injury patterns, and associated health conditions.

However, despite these challenges, substantial progress is being made in the understanding and management of CP as the pace of research efforts in this population has accelerated markedly in recent years. The focus of this article is on the major clinical and theoretical shifts or trends that occurred during the past decade in the medical, surgical, and therapeutic approaches to improving mobility, and more specifically ambulatory abilities, in children with CP. Some of the more dramatic changes in the field have been conceptual and have fundamentally altered how we perceive, classify, and assess a child with CP and how we gauge success of our interventions. New treatments and intervention strategies have also emerged with varying degrees of evidence to support them. Three-dimensional, computer-based analysis of walking and other functional motor tasks has continued to expand the knowledge of normal versus disordered motor control and to quantitatively measure outcomes from interventions designed to improve specific motor skills. Brain and musculoskeletal imaging technologies are also advancing rapidly, and they provide insights into the neuropathology and pathomechanics of CP that were unattainable before their advent.

MAJOR CONCEPTUAL CHANGES IN GOAL SETTING AND CLASSIFICATION OF CP
New Models of Disability

The hallmark of CP is a motor control deficit that differs across individuals in distribution, presentation, and severity. For decades, the direct goal of medical treatment for the motor disability was to alleviate the associated motor impairments, such as spasticity and muscle contracture, with the assumption that functional improvements would ensue. However, that was not necessarily the case,[2] and it was realized that the relationship between impairments and functional activity was neither strong nor linear in many cases.[3] Several conceptual models of disability, most prominently and most recently the World Health Organization's International Classification of Functioning, Disability, and Health (ICF),[4] have shifted the primary focus of treatment to the level of activity and participation of the individual patient. Given family and patient goals in those realms, a treatment plan is proposed and implemented, that may still recommend treatments to address specific impairments in body structures and functions, but could also involve alterations in the environment to improve access or suggestions for family lifestyle changes to increase participation in fitness, sports, or activity-based recreational activities, among other approaches. Many new evaluative measures reflecting these different domains have emerged and are useful in clinical practice and research. The development of parent and child report measures has been particularly notable, and computer-adapted technologies are now being used to obtain comprehensive information in an efficient, user-friendly manner.[5] Although improving activity and participation should be the major treatment priority, interventions that maintain the status quo or minimize future deformity or disability are also beneficial in this population, which may regress in function with time, most dramatically in adulthood.[6]

New and Expanded Classification Schemes

Traditional categorization of subtypes of CP had been based on the primary type of tone disorder and the distribution of the motor involvement, for example, spastic quadriplegia, with each diagnostic category including individuals with a broad range of clinical involvement. The advent of functional classification scales in CP has had a profound effect on determining the prognosis for mobility and related goal setting, improving family and professional communication, and significantly enhancing research design and interpretation. The Gross Motor Functional Classification Scale (GMFCS),[7] which has been adopted universally, categorizes a child's functional mobility ranging from level I, which indicates the highest level of mobility with only minor limitations in more challenging tasks and environments, to level V, which indicates complete dependence on others for mobility. This article primarily addresses those in levels I to –III, who have the capacity or potential for independent, assisted or unassisted, walking. The even more recent Functional Mobility Scale (FMS)[8] expands the assessment of walking ability by rating performance at 3 different distances (5, 50, and 500 meters) that correspond to the 3 major environments that children typically need to navigate: home, school, and the community.

A more global, multiaxial classification scheme for CP[9] has been proposed that encompasses the primary and secondary tone disorders, anatomic distribution of the neurologic involvement, and the functional mobility and upper extremity skill classification, associated impairments, and brain imaging results, yielding a more comprehensive description of the individual patient that should ultimately lead to a more well-focused treatment plan. For example, a child previously categorized as having spastic hemiplegia could now be described in this new classification scheme as having unilateral motor involvement with the presence of both spasticity and dystonia, Manual Ability Classification System[10] level II and GMFCS level I, respectively, with a mild seizure disorder and mild learning deficits, and having MRI evidence of a neonatal stroke.

FACTORS THAT INFLUENCE AMBULATION IN CP, AND THE ROLE OF MEDICAL CARE

Promoting, improving, or restoring the ability to walk is arguably the most common motor goal in neurorehabilitation medicine. Walking status is clearly related to the type and severity of the neurologic deficit, but is not necessarily predetermined by those as illustrated by the conceptual framework of the ICF. It can be influenced in a positive or negative direction by personal factors that may include other associated impairments, as well as emotional, behavioral, and motivational factors. It can also be affected by an individual's physical, social, and cultural environments and the medical care environment, which is the primary focus of this article. In the following 3 sections, the authors summarize the state of the science of medical, surgical, and physical therapy interventions aimed at improving ambulatory function in CP. Although each of these treatment categories are discussed in individual sections, it must be noted that optimal outcomes often depend on the administration of multiple types of interventions administered concurrently or sequentially.

PHYSICAL THERAPY TRENDS FOR AMBULATORY CHILDREN WITH CP

The scientific basis underlying neurologic physical therapy has increased exponentially in the past decade. Before these advances, therapy was dominated by the use of a neurodevelopmental therapy (NDT) approach that has failed to produce consistent clinically significant effects on activity[11] or to demonstrate superiority over alternative approaches.[12] Evidenced-based therapy approaches that are task related and more intense in terms of the amount of practice or effort are being advocated.[13] The use of external devices, such as free weights, weight machines, electrical stimulation units, treadmills, and so on, is also increasingly common in therapy and home programs.

One of the major goals of physical therapy for children with CP in GMFCS levels I to III is to promote independent mobility that includes the ability to ambulate, among other forms of mobility. To accomplish this, children must have adequate active range of motion that is not exceedingly impeded by spasticity, dystonia, or contracture; sufficient strength to maintain body weight support, in some cases with an assistive device; and motor control abilities to allow them to advance their limbs forward to take steps in an effective and efficient manner (eg, minimal scissoring or internal rotation at the hips, minimal crouch in stance, sufficient knee flexion and/or ankle dorsiflexion in swing to allow for foot clearance). The speed and energy costs of walking are also major factors in how functional the gait pattern will be for an individual child. Each of these aspects must be evaluated and addressed by the multidisciplinary team to optimize gait function. Physical therapy can have little, if any, effect on the control of tone abnormalities that require medical and neurosurgical interventions or on the correction of contracture or bony deformity that requires orthopedic surgery; however, it can have a unique and potentially substantial impact on increasing muscle strength and aerobic conditioning and potential in improving lower extremity coordination and speed in this population.

Although stretching is still a component of therapy programs, the use of passive stretching alone has not been shown to be effective,[14] and the impairment of a body structure level goal, such as maintaining muscle length with time, is now more effectively accomplished by interventions such as strength training, dynamic or static orthoses, botulinum toxin (BoNT) injections, or other spasticity-reducing medications or surgeries, although still in combination with manual stretching techniques. As noted above, once a contracture develops, orthopedic surgery to lengthen tendons is often required if the restriction in range impairs function or positioning. Using muscle ultrasound imaging, Shortland and colleagues[15] demonstrated that the fiber lengths of spastic pennated muscles are not necessarily shorter in CP than in age-matched peers, but the length of the aponeurosis is shorter because of decreased fiber diameter resulting from muscle weakness. Their resultant conclusion that strengthening may be a more effective strategy for increasing length in those muscles than stretching runs directly counter to traditional NDT tenets to avoid strengthening or any excessive physical effort so as not to exacerbate spasticity. This long-standing, but unsubstantiated, belief has been increasingly challenged in the literature, and strengthening and other intense activity-based programs are now commonly used in pediatric rehabilitation for children with and without spasticity.[16] Dodd and colleagues[17] conducted a systematic review of the strength training literature in CP. At that time, only 10 research studies met the criteria, which included only 1 randomized controlled trial. Most (8/10) reported significant strength increases as a result of the program. Two studies reported improvements in activity, and 1 study reported improvement in self-perception. No negative effects, such as reduced range of motion or increased spasticity, were reported. Further studies and literature reviews have corroborated these results and similar positive results from programs that involve or include aerobic training.[18–20]

Intense task-specific training has been shown to be effective in several neurologic populations and CP, with the most conclusive findings in CP, demonstrated in intense upper limb training paradigms.[21] For task-specific training in the lower extremity, locomotor training paradigms are commonly used and reported, with many studies incorporating partial body weight–support systems in addition to motorized treadmills. A recent review of the literature on treadmill training in CP[22] demonstrated fairly consistent positive effects on walking speed and the Standing and Walking, Running and Jumping dimensions of the Gross Motor Function Measure. However, no randomized trials that compared treadmill training to over-ground walking of the same intensity have been published to date in CP, even though reviews in stroke and spinal cord suggest that it is the intensity of walking practice, rather than the use of a device, that produces the positive functional outcomes.[23,24] Regardless of whether the results are similar with or without an external device, the use of treadmills and other exercise devices has transformed motor rehabilitation by reinforcing the effectiveness of intense practice, enabling individuals unable to support their own weight to practice walking more easily, and the use of motors and/or added weight support has helped to push people to the limits of their capabilities.[25] Depending on the goal and the exercise protocol designed to accomplish that goal, treadmills can be used to increase strength through progressive loading, increase coordination by training spinal circuits, improve aerobic condition through endurance training, and increase gait speed by progressing belt speeds with time.[26] Thus far, strength and aerobic training and treadmill training programs have been evaluated during short time intervals, but it is important to realize that these are short-term programs in the context of a lifelong disability, and although the effects may be modest, greater functional benefits are likely to accrue with time.[27]

The delivery of physical therapy services has changed dramatically with time, because health insurance in the United States no longer supports the amount of therapy that may be necessary to improve or maintain optimal physical conditioning, with the exception, perhaps, of therapy that follows surgery, which is often more intense. It has now been clearly demonstrated that ambulatory children with CP are far less active than their peers without CP, with the amount of activity directly proportional to their GMFCS level.[28] Decreased activity can lead to loss of strength and increased muscle stiffness, and ultimately to decreased function with time, and it leads to other general health problems in all individuals, with those with motor disabilities being at even greater risk.[29] Physical activity has additionally been shown to contribute positively to mental and emotional functioning.[30,31] Given the changes in health care policy and the recognition that regular and fairly intense physical activity should be part of a daily routine,[32] therapists have been forced to adapt their practices and help families develop other strategies to ensure that their child is as active as possible, in as safe a manner as possible. Identifying activities that are sufficiently physically challenging, enjoyable, or feasible enough to be sustainable and safe for long-term use is a critical element of anticipatory guidance for youth with CP, and to the extent possible, therapists should have input into the design and implementation of these activities. For example, older children may be able to participate in an exercise program at the local YMCA; however, an understanding of their disability and specific impairments is essential in the design of that program, and therapists should be involved in the process to ensure safety and maximum effectiveness. Alternatives to activities that may exacerbate abnormal joint stresses should be considered, such as pool exercises, cycles, or elliptical trainers, in lieu of prolonged treadmill use. For those who are unable to ambulate well outside of the home, adapted and motorized cycles and many over-ground mobility devices are available for recreational or therapeutic use. Beyond the physical and emotional benefits, the importance of activity-based therapies for promoting true neural recovery and restoration in those with brain lesions is just beginning to be realized and is rapidly transforming physical therapy goals and practices.[33]

There has been development of multiple intensive therapy or education-based programs, such as conductive education and Adeli Suit programs, which provide some benefits because of their strong focus on activity and independence, but which also raise some concerns. These programs have failed to demonstrate superior effectiveness over other approaches despite their significantly greater time intensity;[34] they fail to identify the 'active' ingredients, making it hard to determine which aspects of the programs are effective and which are not; they often place additional financial and time constraints on families; and their intensity is not sustainable over the long term, so children may regress when these programs end. Although some of these programs do demonstrate the importance of enhanced training or activity, therapists and the health care system need to ensure that children and families are provided the most effective, time efficient, and preferably community-based therapy programs that are well integrated with other services. To enhance the amount of physical activity and participation, children should be strongly encouraged to participate in self-chosen adapted or regular sports and physical recreational activities. As children transition into later adolescence and adulthood, the responsibility increases for them to establish and maintain their own activity-based goals as part of their own healthy lifestyle choices.

Finally, in addition to the delivery or development of exercise programs, therapists perform many roles that have not been well studied or evaluated scientifically, but are likely to be of critical importance to families and patients and to other members of the multidisciplinary team. As an example, they provide expert advice on how to hold and position a young infant with CP so as to safely promote motor development, they recommend assistive devices to promote mobility, and they may fabricate orthoses or work closely with orthotists and physicians in determining the optimal type of orthosis for an individual patient depending on his/her abilities and goals. Therapists are often a major source of medical information to the family and, because of their regular contact with the child and family, they may often be the first to recognize the potential need for other treatments and may work with the family in communicating with or identifying a physician or surgeon who will evaluate the child for other interventions.

MEDICAL MANAGEMENT OF MOTOR DISORDERS IN AMBULATORY PATIENTS WITH CP
Overview of Recent Changes in the Approach to Diagnosis and Treatment

CP is a group of disorders of movement and posture with varying causes.[35] As the knowledge of specific neurologic disorders has expanded, more of the specific causes of motor and movement disorders in children, such as hereditary dystonias and the ever-expanding group of mitochondrial disorders,[36–38] can be potentially identified. Whether these disorders should be grouped with the cerebral palsies remains unclear. In the future, identifying specific disorders will be increasingly important as specialized treatments for these conditions become available.

Patients with CP present with both positive and negative features of the upper motor neuron syndrome at the level of body structures and functions in the ICF model.[39–41] These include a variety of tone abnormalities ranging from hypotonia to hyperkinesis. Because patients with CP were traditionally classified by their predominant tone abnormality, that is, spasticity or dyskinesis, the nuances of mixed tone disorders were often missed. Selective, specific therapies[38] increase the importance of correctly identifying mixed patterns of abnormal tone. For example, a patient with mixed spastic dyskinetic CP is not a good candidate for selective dorsal rhizotomy (SDR), but may be a candidate for intrathecal baclofen therapy (ITB). Mixed tone disorders require a more studied approach when considering treatment options.[42]

In the past, the selection of medical treatment for motor disorders associated with CP often started with what was viewed as less invasive treatment, later moving to more invasive interventions. This hierarchical model has largely been replaced by an integrated model where several interventions are used in series, or often concurrently, and at various times throughout a patient's life. For ambulatory patients with CP, several treatment modalities may be selected at the same time. For example, BoNT to address focal tone issues such as an equinus foot or flexed knee may be combined with physical therapy to strengthen the antagonist and maximize function, with orthoses to provide additional stretch, and with oral medications at night or during the day to reduce spasms.[43,44] This integrated treatment approach is often provided by an interdisciplinary health care team of physicians and therapists. In the 21st century, few clinicians work in isolation when providing care for patients with CP.[45] Most pediatric hospitals and clinics provide interdisciplinary care in one form or another, although the composition of the team and its functional model varies widely across institutions. Team models range from structured programs to a loose affiliation of clinicians who communicate by e-mail, telephone, or written records. Even when located in remote locations, many clinicians now have access to the Internet and can thereby contact colleagues with whom they may consult. This enhanced communication has fundamentally transformed the relationships among individuals from differing disciplines and the way care is delivered to patients. Enhanced communication among medical, rehabilitation, and surgical specialists has increased the knowledge of all practitioners involved in the team, with patients as the ultimate beneficiaries of resultant improved care and coordination.[46–48]

Interdisciplinary teams have also moved towards incorporating evidence-based medicine into daily practice, no longer relying solely on past or anecdotal experience to make decisions about care for individuals with CP. Future studies must critically evaluate the short- and long-term impact of treatment effects on function and quality of life. In the past, most studies focused on impairments instead of function or participation. There have now been a number of studies evaluating the functional efficacy of BoNT therapy, SDR, and ITB.[49,50] To date, only few oral medication studies have evaluated effects of treatment on function or participation.[38,51] It is critical for future studies of medical management techniques to incorporate functional assessment in outcome data. Key to this evaluation is to develop outcome tools that are meaningful and are sensitive to change and to prescribe only those interventions that provide clinically important changes in patient function.

Rationale for Treatment Selection

Recent years have seen a greater focus on 'tone management', primarily to minimize the development of contractures and facilitate ease of movement. An increasing array of medical treatment options, including medications, biologic agents, and surgical interventions, are available for management of abnormal muscle tone in patients with CP.[43,52,53] A thorough understanding of neurophysiology and pharmacology is required to guide clinicians in selecting the most appropriate medications or agents. Although often requested, there are no medical treatments that ameliorate other impairments associated with CP, that is, weakness, balance, and motor control. Other factors affecting patient function and participation include patient motivation, family commitment, social support, access to intervention/treatment, and geographic location. Clinicians must consider all of these issues when selecting from available treatment options and interventions.

Medical management of the motor disorders in children with CP is most often provided by 1 or more physicians, including physiatrists, neurologists, developmental pediatricians, and orthopedists. One of the first decisions for physicians is to determine whether treatment or intervention is needed. Not all abnormal tone is harmful. There may be benefits to increased tone, including preserved skeletal and muscle mass, decreased edema, aiding standing and transfers, prevention of decubiti, and reduced deep vein thrombosis risks.[40] Treatment should only be initiated if the abnormal tone is symptomatic. The next decision is when to initiate treatment. Medical interventions may be initiated in infancy if deemed necessary. This decision is based on a detailed clinical assessment, review of therapy notes, and evaluation of the patient's impairments, body structures (passive range of motion [PROM], active range of motion), and functional capabilities.[54] Physicians must evaluate/observe patients as they perform functional activities to identify problem muscles and work with them to establish treatment goals. The physical therapist or occupational therapist treating a patient weekly may identify different problems/goals than the MD who sees a patient quarterly. Input from each member of the team is critical to the decision-making process.[55]

Once problematic muscle tone has been identified, the next step is to determine the choice of intervention or interventions from among the many options available. Options include oral medications and injectable agents (BoNT, phenol, alcohol). ITB therapy, SDR, and deep brain stimulation are tone-reducing treatments that require surgical intervention.[43,44,53] Once the pump is implanted, however, ITB becomes a medical intervention.[56] These and other interventions are often performed in series or in combination during the course of a patient's life.

Complementary and alternative medicine (CAM) may also be recommended by physicians or chosen by families. CAM options for treating patients with CP include acupuncture, massage, homeopathic remedies, herbal treatments, and magnet therapy, to list a few, each with varying degrees of evidence available. It is important for clinicians to ask about use of these treatments, particularly herbal medications, as these may interact with prescribed medications.

Treatment of abnormal tone is frequently initiated to facilitate other interventions, such as therapy, casting, and bracing/splinting. Medical treatment is continually revised and continued as needed, based on review of clinical and functional goals set by the team, patient, and family. Medical therapy is directed toward improving symptoms, not only at the impairment level, but also at the level of improving function. Functional goals as defined by Mayer and colleagues[57] include passive function (functional activities that happen to the patient, such as hygiene or dressing) or active function (activities that the patients perform for themselves). Decisions regarding when to begin, change, or stop medical therapy are based on short- and long-term treatment goals and responses to treatment.

Many clinicians advocate BoNT therapy as the initial treatment for young ambulatory children with CP and problematic focal spasticity or dystonia. The goals of early BoNT treatment include preserving PROM/ prevention of contractures, facilitating therapy, improving mobility/gait, and delaying orthopedic surgery. Other treatment options, including oral medications, are added as needed, based on response to BoNT treatment and treatment goals. A bedtime dose of valium or baclofen may be added to the treatment plan to decrease spasms or pain and increase compliance with nighttime splinting. BoNT therapy is often recommended throughout early childhood. Continued treatment is based on a patient's response to BoNT therapy and treatment goals. Oral medications are less frequently used during the day due to central nervous system (CNS) side effects, including sedation, impaired learning, and other cognitive side effects, but are appropriate for some children with CP, with or without BoNT. Because of dosing limitations with BoNT treatment, this may be combined with phenol or alcohol blocks (eg, obturator nerve block for adductor tone/ scissoring in ambulatory patients) to allow a greater number of muscles to be treated than if BoNT was used alone.[43,44,58-64]

Efficacy of BoNT requires accurate placement of the toxin within the target muscle(s). A variety of approaches are used, including anatomic guidance/palpation, electromyography (EMG), and electrical stimulation. Ultrasound has been used for decades to guide biopsies and procedures. Advances in high frequency transducer technology have led to an explosion of ultrasound use in musculoskeletal imaging, including guidance for BoNT therapy. Ultrasound allows the painless, accurate identification of target muscles and is therefore frequently preferred by patients over other localization techniques. Other advantages cited are increased ease of identifying deep muscles or muscles with overlapping anatomy, reduction of administration time, and lack of requirement for the larger needles in comparison to the EMG-guided technique.[65–68]

Although better spasticity management is purportedly diminishing the need for future orthopedic surgery,[69] many children who initially benefit from BoNT therapy later require orthopedic surgery[70] (see following surgical section). BoNT may be provided before muscle lengthening, osteotomy, or single event multilevel surgery. This perioperative treatment has been shown to reduce muscle spasm, postoperative pain, length of stay, and use of pain medication.[71] Some clinicians continue to advocate BoNT therapy throughout a patient's lifespan. Treatment is often reinitiated during accelerated teen growth to address increased dynamic tone, ROM limitations, and changes in gait. BoNT therapy in ambulatory adult patients may also be helpful in preserving ROM, gait, and mobility and in reducing pain.

Based on regular reevaluation of symptoms, impairments, and function, a patient's medical treatment is continually modified. In some centers, SDR is frequently recommended for ambulatory patients with spastic CP. This is most often performed between the ages of 4 and 8. Some clinicians advocate performing orthopedic procedures first and then reevaluating the patient's function before proceeding with SDR, whereas others favor spasticity intervention first. There are no guidelines in the literature to support one algorithm over the other. Functional improvement after SDR is highly dependent on patient selection. Comprehensive, interdisciplinary evaluation is essential, including evaluation of strength, motor control, and mobility. In many centers, ITB is used most frequently in nonambulatory patients (GMFCS levels IV–V). Other centers advocate ITB to improve ambulation in patients with CP. In studies with careful selection criteria, improved long-term ambulation in patients receiving ITB is supported by the literature.[72–77]

REVIEW OF NEUROANATOMIC AND NEUROPHYSIOLOGIC ISSUES INFLUENCING TREATMENT OF MOTOR DISORDERS ASSOCIATED WITH CP

Medical intervention requires a basic understanding of the neurophysiology underlying the maintenance of normal tone, which involves the complex interaction of many structures and pathways within the CNS. The pyramidal and extrapyramidal systems are involved in generating positive and inhibitory descending signals to the spinal cord and alpha motor neuron. Lesions at any site along these pathways can disrupt the normal balance between excitation and inhibition. Pharmacologic treatments may be directed at structures within the CNS, the peripheral nerve, neuromuscular junction, or directly at the muscle itself. Medications with mechanisms of action (MOAs) on the CNS include drugs or modalities that modulate/change descending inhibitory signals, reduce the release of excitatory neurotransmitters, or modulate spinal cord reflex pathways involved in abnormal tone or spasticity.

Definitions of Tone Disorders

Spasticity is characterized by resistance to stretch and may be either or both velocity- and position-dependent. It results from CNS pathology leading to loss of descending inhibition, often in the pyramidal tracts. Loss of presynaptic inhibitory signals results in decreased synthesis or transport of GABA to the anterior horn cell. This leads to altered synaptic input and membrane properties and results in hyperexcitability of the alpha motor neuron. Severe spasticity often masks underlying movement disorders or dystonia. Careful clinical assessment should be done in varied settings and positions, with different velocities.[78–81]

Dystonia is characterized by sustained muscle contractions or postures, often twisting or repetitive in nature. Classically, dystonia presents with co-contraction of agonist and antagonist muscles as a result of failed reciprocal inhibition. Overflow or spread to proximal and distal muscles and other regions commonly occurs. Some patients may present with dystonic posturing only with activity, whereas in other patients dystonia may be present at rest. Injury to the brainstem, basal ganglia, and thalamus affects GABA synthesis or transport, leading to dystonia and other movement disorders. Normally the basal ganglia provide the memory for controlled or skilled movements.[38,82,83] The thalamus creates a zone of inhibition, modulating descending signals from the motor cortex. When this is damaged, the modulating effects of the basal ganglia are disrupted, leading to abnormal tone and movement patterns. In patients who have CP, dystonia may not be evident until a child is nearly 3 years or older, because of continuing brain reorganization and maturation. Inherited forms of dystonia also may present in childhood, such as dopamine-responsive dystonia (DRD). DRD should be considered in any patient presenting with dystonia and CP, particularly when there is diurnal variation in symptoms, dystonia is progressive, and the lower extremities are preferentially involved.[36,38] Symptoms of DRD vary widely at onset and may mimic motor symptoms of CP. Nygaard and colleagues[36] estimated that 5% to 10% of patients presenting with pediatric onset dystonia actually have DRD. Given the inherited nature of DRD, obtaining a detailed family history is critical. A trial of dopamine may be indicated in most, if not all, patients presenting with dystonic CP to clinically rule out a DRD.

Hyperkinetic disorders include chorea, athetosis, choreoathetosis, ballism, tics, myoclonus, stereotypies, and rigidity. These disorders are less well described than spasticity and dystonia. A pediatric Movement Disorders Taskforce, funded by the NIH, has convened for several years to develop or revise descriptors for each of these disorders to more clearly differentiate them. The final document with these descriptors is pending publication.Treatment options available at present are more limited than those for spasticity.

Pharmacology of Medication Management of Tone Disorders

Medications may influence abnormal tone by modulating input to or output from a variety of sites within or outside the CNS, including higher cortical centers, the basal ganglia, cerebellum, spinal cord, and muscle. The neurons and interneurons influenced by medications use a variety of neurotransmitters, including epinephrine, norepinephrine, serotonin, GABA, glutamate, glutamine, dopamine, and substance P, among others. Descending pathways that may be influenced by medications are described in more detail in **Fig. 1**. **Table 1** summarizes the primary function of each pathway. Medications can act at numerous sites and pathways in the CNS, at the neuromuscular junction, and on muscle. Most centrally acting medications work by altering release of excitatory neurotransmitters or increasing inhibitory neurotransmitter release. Peripheral sites of action include the neuromuscular junction, nerve, and muscle. Phenol and alcohol demyelinate motor nerves, reducing stimulation of the muscle. Neurotoxins reduce presynaptic release of acetylcholine at the neuromuscular junction, thereby decreasing muscle stimulation. There is only 1 drug with an

NEUROTRANSMITTER	Excitatory							Inhibitory		
PATHWAY/STURCTURES	Glut	Dopa	Epi	Nor-Epi	SRT	Sub P	Exteroceptive /Sensory	GABA	GLY	α – adren
Cortical	+		+	+				++	+	+
Brain Stem		+						++	+	
Corticospinal	+++		+	+				++	+	
Locus Ceruleus	+							++	+	++
Reticulospinal				+++	+++			++	+	
Vestibulospinal								++	+	
Spinal cord	++		+	+		++	++	++	+	++

Fig. 1. Known or expected effects of specific neurotransmitters on neural structures or pathways. *Abbreviations:* α–adren, alpha adrenergic; dopa, dopamine; epi, epinephrine; GABA, gamma aminobutyric acid; GLUT, glutamate; GLY, glycerine; nor-epi, norepinepherine; sensory/exteroceptive, sensory signals from outside CNS; SRT, serotonin; subP, substance P.

MOA having direct effect on the muscle. Dantrolene sodium interferes with the release of calcium from the sarcoplasmic reticulum, thereby decreasing excitation/contraction coupling and the force of muscle contraction.

MEDICATIONS FOR SPASTICITY AND DYSTONIA

The MOA of most medications is incompletely understood. Multiple sites of action within the CNS are possible. Variability in efficacy, response, dosing, and side effects in individual patients must be considered the norm and not the exception. Recognizing this variability is critical in evaluating medication effectiveness and dosing in an individual patient. It is estimated that only 30% of patients have a positive response to oral medications. To date, there is little level 1 evidence to support use of one medication over another. In addition, few studies have evaluated the effect of medications on function. The use of medications is often driven by clinician experience and training, patient age, side-effect profile, and distribution/severity of the tone disorder.

Selecting Medications and Treatment for a Patient

Oral medications and/or ITB are generally used for patients who have generalized and/ or severe spasticity or dystonia. Injectable medications and agents such as phenol/ alcohol and the BoNTs are used most often for focal, multifocal, and regional tone disorders. Combined treatment with oral medications or ITB and injectable agents is often used in patients with generalized tone disorders with focal deficits limiting function or comfort. An example of this would be the use of BoNT to address upper extremity spasticity in patients whose upper extremity tone is incompletely controlled by ITB. BoNTs and oral medications may also be used together to supplement efficacy of the individual agents and prevent side effects of high doses of oral medications. **Table 2** provides a list, expanded in recent years, of medications that have been used in patients treated for abnormal muscle tone. The evidence for effective use of many of these medications is from the adult literature. The evidence to support use of these medications in pediatrics is primarily based on anecdotal experience. Obtaining approval for placebo-controlled medication trials in children is complicated by the difficulty in obtaining informed consent in minors. Supported by the Best Pharmaceuticals for Children Act, which mandates testing for pediatric medications on children, models that would expand pediatric drug testing are now being explored and

Table 1
The major function or action of specific brain areas or pathways

Structure/ Pathway	Brainstem	Pyramidal/ Corticospinal Pathways	Reticulospinal Pathways	Vestibulospinal Pathways	Locus Ceruleus	Spinal Cord	NMJ/ Muscle
Function or action	Modulates: cortical signals/ motor plan. Closed loop contact with cortex. No direct descending output to spinal cord	Discrete distal extremity-controlled movements	Trunk and proximal extremity control and posture	Head/trunk control, position in space	Facilitatory drive to spinal cord and spinal pathways	Net balance: facilitation and inhibition leads to increased or decreased signals/drive to α MN	α MN drive leads to release of ACH and muscle contraction

Abbreviations: ACH, acetylcholine; α MN, alpha motor neuron; NMJ, neuromuscular junction.

Table 2
The most common (primary) and less common (secondary) medications for the major disorders of tone and movement in cerebral palsy

Spasticity medications		
Primary	**Secondary**	
Benzodiazepines	Cyproheptadine	Clorazepate
Baclofen	Clonidine	Ketazolam
Dantrolene	Lamotrigine	Piracetam
Tizanidine	Tiagabine	Progabide
Botulinum toxins	Gabapentin	Orphenadrine
Phenol/alcohol	Pregabalin	Cannaboids
Dystonia medications		
Primary	**Secondary**	
Dopaminergic therapy	Calcium channel blockers	
Levodopa/carbidopa	Antidopaminergic drugs	
Anticholinergics	Tizanadine	
Trihexyphenidyl	Clonazepam	
Baclofen	Tetrabenazine	

implemented. In future medication trials, incorporating evaluation of functional outcomes is imperative.

The above medications have varying efficacy, MOAs, and side-effect profiles. Prescribing physicians must be familiar with the medication's interactions and need for drug monitoring. Selection of medications must include consideration of the patient's clinical indications and comorbidities. No 1 treatment or medication is effective for a specific tone disorder or group of patients. Selecting medications is an art, based on the science to support use of the medication and the patient's motor disability.

ORTHOPEDIC MANAGEMENT OF MOTOR DISORDERS IN CP

In the 1800s, William Little, a surgeon from England, began using the technique of percutaneous Achilles tenotomy (transecting the tendon) to treat children and adults with paralytic foot deformities, such as those with CP. In fact, the name for CP used until even recently was "Little's disease." There was little improvement on the technique of tenotomy or other musculotendinous surgery until the polio epidemic, when many different tendon lengthenings and transfers were developed, and the field of orthopedics blossomed. With the decline in polio, orthopedic surgeons turned their attention to other neuromuscular diseases, such as myelomeningocele and CP.

Based on the experience of the polio epidemic, in which only 1 or a few motor levels were affected, surgeons began operating on 1 joint at a time.[84,85] For example, a child who was walking on his toes and had a flexion contracture at his hips and knees would have a heel cord lengthening, then the next year, a distal hamstring lengthening, and the next year, a hip flexor lengthening. Mercer Rang called this the "birthday syndrome," in which the child was in the hospital every year of his life getting an operation. This has been shown to be an unwise approach to surgery for patients with CP. The best outcomes occur in those children who have single event-multilevel surgery (SEMLS) with physical therapy and appropriate (usually ankle-foot orthoses) bracing.[86,87] This can involve performing bony osteotomies to correct rotational problems combined with tendon lengthening and transfers at the hip, knee, and ankle at the same operative procedure.

The indications to perform orthopedic surgery on children with CP are to improve function, prevent deformity, decrease pain from joint dislocation or subluxation, prevent skin pressure areas, improve sitting position, improve cosmesis and hygiene, and facilitate orthotic management.[88,89] In all cases, the surgeon should work closely with a team that might include physical and occupational therapists, neurologists, and physiatrists. There should be consensus on the best treatment plan. For example, the child may be an ambulator who has a combination of spasticity and dystonia, but primarily spasticity. The physiatrist may recommend a course of oral antispasticity medication, perhaps chemodenervation of the nerve or phenol injections to the motor nerves before surgery or in conjunction with the surgery. It might be suggested that surgery be delayed for several months to years, with interim use of physical therapeutic modalities and casting. A critical part of any surgery is the postoperative rehabilitation, including appropriate bracing, strengthening, and gait training. In those children who are undergoing hip reduction surgery, the wheelchair seating system often does not fit correctly postoperatively and this must be anticipated preoperatively.

The introduction of the GMFCS and the FMS has significantly impacted orthopedic surgeons' thinking. Surgeries designed to improve ambulation are preferred in patients at levels GMFCS II and III, whereas operations to permit pain-free sitting are performed for those at levels GMFCS IV and V.[7,8] It is clear that those patients who have more involvement (levels IV and V) have more dystonia and mixed motor patterns. Therefore, therapies aimed at reducing these movement problems should be implemented concurrently with any planned orthopedic surgery. The GMFCS level can also play a role in deciding whether a child should have a screening radiograph for hip dysplasia. Hagglund and colleagues[90] found that a child with GMFCS I had a 0% chance of having hip dislocation, whereas a child with GMFCS V had a 64% chance.

Orthopedic surgery does not affect motor control and balance or improve muscular strength.[91] It may have a short-term effect on spasticity as the muscular tension is altered, which affects the Golgi tendon apparatus and the muscle spindle. However, as noted in the section on spasticity management, the orthopedic surgeon is a member of a team that addresses spasticity management and pre- and postoperative rehabilitation. Boyd and Graham suggested a treatment algorithm in which orthopedic surgery is delayed until about age 7 to 9 years, with a greater focus on physical therapy and spasticity management in the early years. The major exception to that would be if the hip is coming out of the joint, secondary to muscle contractures.[92] This delay in surgical intervention has several advantages, such as allowing more development of the musculoskeletal system; permitting a "declaration" of the movement disorder, because it is sometimes difficult to distinguish between severe spasticity and dystonia in the very young child; and allowing studies such as gait laboratory evaluation to enable SEMLS. Although the long-term effect of this algorithm is still being studied, the hypothesis that fewer orthopedic surgeries and ultimately better long-term function will be observed is likely correct in patients treated in this manner.

Technology has also had a major impact in the preoperative planning for orthopedic surgery on the lower extremity. In some of the most advanced centers, 3-dimensional gait analysis is used to completely evaluate the motion at each of the joints in the lower extremities, the forces that cross each joint, and when the muscles fire based on dynamic EMG. Energy utilization is 1 measure to evaluate the impact of different therapies on the child preoperatively and postoperatively. Although there is contro-versy as to the clinical usefulness of gait analysis, there is no question that it can be a critical tool to evaluate novel surgeries and the outcomes of therapy. Many experi-enced orthopedic surgeons who operate on children with CP often rely on these data to plan their surgery.

Computer modeling using cadaver-derived models coupled with gait analysis data from actual patients is an important research tool and a method to gain insight into complex biologic problems. These models may enable determination whether a partic-ular surgery would lead to the anticipated results. Delp and his research teams[94] have been leaders in this field and have provided many thought-provoking articles in this arena. There have been several excellent studies using computer models to replicate the anatomy and muscle activity about the hip, ranging from evaluation of "internal rotation" gait and its treatment,[93] the effect of hip flexion on moment arms,[94] and the effect of flexion in crouch gait on hip extension.[95] This basic science tool has certainly improved the understanding of the biomechanical forces, but as yet it has not been used to provide individualized treatment plans for actual patients, which is the hope and promise of this technology.

Orthopedic surgery should be considered in children if they have significant fixed contractures of their joints; if there is a subluxation or dislocation of a joint, particularly the hip joint; if there are rotational problems that cause walking problems; if there is curvature of the spine that impacts the child's sitting or might be anticipated to cause pulmonary problems as the child ages; or if there are hygiene or pain problems secondary to any of the above. Pain is usually not present in young children, but it can be a significant problem as the patients become young adults. Knowledge of the natural history of CP may lead the surgeon to suggest surgery even when there does not appear to be a significant problem, such as pes valgus, hip subluxation, or early scoliosis.

There are basically 4 major types of orthopedic surgery performed in children with CP:

- Musculotendinous or tendon lengthenings
- Tendon transfers
- Osteotomies
- Arthrodeses

Peripheral neurectomy may be performed, although the long-term outcome is not predictable and this is not routinely performed.

Musculotendinous Lengthening

This is a surgery that involves a lengthening of the musculotendinous unit. The tendon can be lengthened in a Z-type fashion (**Fig. 2**)[96] or at the musculotendinous junction or through the fascia as a recession (**Fig. 3**).[96,97] Simple tenotomies (transecting the tendon) often have poor outcomes, although they have a place in hip adductor surgery.

This procedure is indicated when a contracture is present, that is, the joint that the muscle crosses cannot be moved passively through the full range. There is some decrease in spasticity after tendon lengthening, most likely because of an alteration of the Golgi receptors and muscle spindles in the muscle. Complications include over-lengthening of the tendon (usually iatrogenic) and weakness.[98] Recent research suggests that the tendon may actually be long, but the muscle fibers are shortened, so lengthening of the tendon may be deleterious to the muscle (see earlier section).

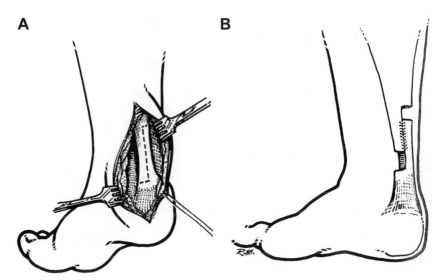

Fig. 2. Tendon Achilles lengthening procedure showing the intact (*A*) and resutured (*B*) tendon. (*From* Canale ST, Beaty JH. Operative pediatric orthopedics. St Louis: Mosby–Year Book; 1991. p. 664; with permission.)

Tendon Transfers

In CP, tendon transfers are used to take a muscle that is spastic and contributing to a deformity and repositioning it (or part of it) to perform another function. The muscle may then be used to balance a joint or even to serve as a functional transfer.

In the upper extremity, a common transfer in CP is the Green transfer, in which the flexor carpi ulnaris muscle (which serves to flex and ulnarly deviate the wrist) is transferred to the dorsum of the wrist to serve as a wrist extensor and radial deviator. A modification of this technique has been described, in which the flexor carpi ulnaris is transferred to the common finger extensors to allow for extension of the fingers and facilitation of release of objects in the hand.[99,100] Other procedures have been devised to improve the position and the function of the hand and fingers.[101]

In the lower extremity, several transfers have been used to improve function. In patients with a stiff-knee gait, transfer of the rectus femoris muscle to the hamstrings has been shown to improve the knee range of motion and gait, particularly swing phase clearance of the foot.[102] In patients with spastic hemiplegia and a varus foot deformity, a split transfer of the tibialis anterior or tibialis posterior muscle can correct the position of the foot to neutral.[103]

Osteotomies

If left untreated, the action of the spastic muscles can lead to deformity of the bones and alteration of the joint mechanics (subluxation or dislocation). In some ambulatory children, rotational abnormalities (increased femoral anteversion and internal or external tibial torsion) can lead to "lever-arm disease."[104–106] All children are born with increased femoral anteversion, but normal ambulation leads to a natural derotation of the femur. This may fail to occur in CP and may need to be corrected, if the muscles are to work in their normal biomechanical alignment. The use of osteotomies, including shortening osteotomies, has decreased the use of tendon lengthening and is preferred by some orthopedists when possible.

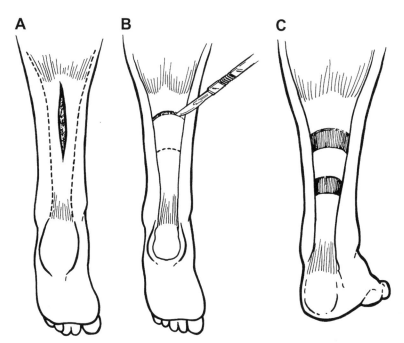

Fig. 3. Gastroc-soleus recession procedure that only lengthens the uppermost gastrocnemius portion of the tendon. (*From* Canale ST, Beaty JH. Operative pediatric orthopedics. St Louis: Mosby–Year Book; 1991. p. 664; with permission.)

In primarily marginal or nonambulatory children, the hip joint can dislocate, causing seating problems and eventually arthritis and pain. In these cases, surgery aimed at reducing the hips and preventing further dislocation is performed.[106–111]

Children with CP may develop multiple deformities at the foot and ankle, which may prevent or limit ambulation and occasionally even the wearing of normal shoes. Multiple osteotomies of the tibia and fibula and all of the bones of the foot have been developed to more correctly align the foot.

Arthrodeses

In some cases, arthrodesis, or fusion of the joints, is necessary to place the joint in an optimum position. Fusion of the hip is rarely warranted because of the difficulty in sitting and/or standing after the fusion. Very good results have been obtained in fusion of the thumb and wrist. The best results in fusion in CP include arthrodesis of the first metatarsal phalangeal joint of the hallux.[112] So-called extraarticular fusions of the foot for valgus deformity, such as Grice or Green procedures, are still used to help stabilize the foot, but other newer procedures, such as a calcaneal lengthening osteotomy, have supplanted this as the preferred treatment of the spastic valgus foot.[113,114] The most common arthrodesis is a spine fusion to treat the scoliosis that children with spastic quadriplegia often develop.[115]

Insummary, orthopedic surgery has an important role in the management of children and adults with CP. Clinicians should strive to control spasticity, in conjunction with musculotendinous and bony surgery, to maximize each other's gains. A team approach with physicians, nurses, and physical, occupational, and speech therapists working together with that patient and family with careful, predetermined goals will serve the patient's needs and aspirations.

SUMMARY

When treating children with CP, clinicians need to be constantly asking themselves the question: what can we be doing in childhood, or what should we not be doing, to maximize mobility and independence in adulthood? It is critical that individuals with CP are helped to contiue to maintain the physical capabilities that they have through targeted tone management, joint-friendly exercise strategies, and the judicious use of surgeries that reduce muscle force production or sensory input. More well-informed application of principles of biomechanics, exercise physiology, and motor control to this population and new knowledge of mechanisms underlying neural recovery and restoration are transforming the scientific basis of intervention strategies. More accurate diagnoses, new developments in prevention of primary and secondary impairments, and technological advances in brain and body imaging and in rehabilitation device design also have great promise and potential for improving outcomes in terms of health status and, most importantly, the quality of life for individuals with CP.

REFERENCES

1. Yeargin-Allsopp M, Van Naarden Braun K, Doernberg NS, et al. Prevalence of cerebral palsy in 8-year-old children in three areas of the United States in 2002: a multisite collaboration. Pediatrics 2008;121:547–54.
2. Sahrmann SA, Norton BJ. The relationship of voluntary movement to spasticity in the upper motor neuron syndrome. Ann Neurol 1977;2:460–5.
3. Abel MF, Damiano DL, Blanco JS, et al. Relationships among musculoskeletal impairments and functional health status in ambulatory cerebral palsy. J Pediatr Orthop 2003;23:535–41.
4. World Health Organization. International classification of functioning, disability, and health. World Health Organization; 2001.
5. Haley SM, Raczek AE, Coster WJ, et al. Assessing mobility in children using a computer adaptive testing version of the pediatric evaluation of disability inventory. Arch Phys Med Rehabil 2005;86:932–9.
6. Bottos M, Gericke C. Ambulatory capacity in cerebral palsy: prognostic criteria and consequences for intervention. Dev Med Child Neurol 2003;45:786–90.
7. Rosenbaum PL, Palisano RJ, Bartlett DJ, et al. Development of the gross motor function classification system for cerebral palsy. Dev Med Child Neurol 2008;50:249–53.
8. Graham HK, Harvey A, Rodda J, et al. The Functional Mobility Scale (FMS). J Pediatr Orthop 2004;24:514–20.
9. Rosenbaum P, Paneth N, Leviton A, et al. A report: the definition and classification of cerebral palsy April 2006. Dev Med Child Neurol Suppl 2007;109:8–14.
10. Eliasson AC, Krumlinde-Sundholm L, Rösblad B, et al. The Manual Ability Classification System (MACS) for children with cerebral palsy: scale development and evidence of validity and reliability. Dev Med Child Neurol 2006;48:549–54.
11. Knox V, Evans AL. Evaluation of the functional effects of a course of Bobath therapy in children with cerebral palsy: a preliminary study. Dev Med Child Neurol 2002;44:447–60.
12. Butler C, Darrah J. Effects of neurodevelopmental treatment (NDT) for cerebral palsy: an AACPDM evidence report. Dev Med Child Neurol 2001;43:778–90.
13. Crompton J, Imms C, McCoy AT, et al. Group-based task-related training for children with cerebral palsy: a pilot study. Phys Occup Ther Pediatr 2007;27:43–65.

14. Wiart L, Darrah J, Kembhavi G. Stretching with children with cerebral palsy: what do we know and where are we going? Pediatr Phys Ther 2008;20:173–8.

15. Shortland AP, Harris CA, Gough M, et al. Architecture of the medial gastrocnemius in children with spastic diplegia. Dev Med Child Neurol 2002;44:158–63.

16. Damiano DL. Activity, activity, activity: rethinking our physical therapy approach to cerebral palsy. Phys Ther 2006;86:1534–40.

17. Dodd K, Taylor N, Damiano DL. A systematic review of the effectiveness of strength-training programs for people with cerebral palsy. Arch Phys Med Rehabil 2002;83:1157–64.

18. Mockford M, Caulton JM. Systematic review of progressive strength training in children and adolescents with cerebral palsy who are ambulatory. Pediatr Phys Ther 2008;20:318–33.

19. Verschuren O, Ketelaar M, Takken T, et al. Exercise programs for children with cerebral palsy: a systematic review of the literature. Am J Phys Med Rehabil 2008;87:404–17.

20. Rogers A, Furler BL, Brinks S, et al. A systematic review of the effectiveness of aerobic exercise interventions for children with cerebral palsy: an AACPDM evidence report. Dev Med Child Neurol 2008;50:808–14.

21. Hoare BJ, Wasiak J, Imms C, et al. Constraint-induced movement therapy in the treatment of the upper limb in children with hemiplegic cerebral palsy. Cochrane Database Syst Rev 2007;18:CD004149.

22. Damiano DL, DeJong SL. A systematic review of the effects of treadmill training and body weight support in pediatric rehabilitation. J Neurol Phys Ther 2009;33(1):27–44.

23. Eng JJ, Tang PF. Gait training strategies to optimize walking ability in people with stroke: a synthesis of the evidence. Expert Rev Neurother 2007;7(10):1417–36.

24. Mehrholz J, Kugler J, Pohl M. Locomotor training for walking after spinal cord injury. Cochrane Database Syst Rev 2008 Apr 16;(2):CD006676.

25. Hesse S. Treadmill training with partial body weight support after stroke: a review. NeuroRehabilitation 2008;23:55–65.

26. Cernak K, Stevens V, Price R, et al. Locomotor training using body-weight support on a treadmill in conjunction with ongoing physical therapy in a child with severe cerebellar ataxia. Phys Ther 2008;88:88–97.

27. Taylor N, Dodd KJ, Damiano DL. Progressive resistance exercise in physical therapy: a summary of systematic reviews. Phys Ther 2005;85:1208–23.

28. Bjornson KF, Belza B, Kartin D, et al. Ambulatory physical activity performance in youth with cerebral palsy and youth who are developing typically. Phys Ther 2007;87:248–57.

29. Durstine JL, Painter P, Franklin BA, et al. Physical activity for the chronically ill and disabled. Sports Med 2000;30(3):207–19.

30. van Uffelen JG, Chin A Paw MJ, Hopman-Rock M, et al. The effects of exercise on cognition in older adults with and without cognitive decline: a systematic review. Clin J Sport Med 2008;18:486–500.

31. Ströhle A. Physical activity, exercise, depression and anxiety disorders. J Neural Transm 2008; Aug 23 [Epub ahead of print].

32. Morris PJ. Physical activity recommendations for children and adolescents with chronic disease. Curr Sports Med Rep 2008;7:353–8.

33. Behrman AL, Bowden MG, Nair PM. Neuroplasticity after spinal cord injury and training: an emerging paradigm shift in rehabilitation and walking recovery. Phys Ther 2006;86:1406–25.

34. Anttila H, Suoranta J, Malmivaara A, et al. Effectiveness of physiotherapy and conductive education interventions in children with cerebral palsy: a focused review. Am J Phys Med Rehabil 2008;87:478–501.

35. O'Shea TM. Diagnosis treatment, and prevention of cerebral palsy. Clin Obstet Gynecol 2008;51(4):816–28.

36. Nygaard TG, Marsden CD, Duvoisin RC. Dopa-responsive dystonia. Adv Neurol 1988;50:377–84.

37. Bressman SB, Tagliati M, Klein C. Genetics of dystonia. Dystonia: etiology, clinical features, and treatment. WE MOVE; 2004. p. 11–21. Available at: http://www.wemove.org. Accessed April 28, 2009.

38. Bhidayasiri R, Tarsy D. Treatment of dystonia. Expert Rev Neurother 2006;6:863–86.

39. Mayer NH. Spasticity and the stretch reflex. Muscle Nerve 1997;20(Suppl 6):S1–3.

40. Mayer NH, Herman RM. Positive signs and consequences of an upper motor neuron syndrome. Spasticity and other forms of muscle over activity in the upper motor neuron syndrome. WE MOVE; p. 11–26. Available at: http://www.wemove.org. Accessed April 28, 2009.

41. Gracies JM, Elovic E, Nance P. Traditional pharmacological treatment for spasticity part II. Muscle Nerve 1997;6:S92–120.

42. Adam OR, Jankovic J. Treatment of dystonia disorders [review]. Parkinsonism Relat Disord 2007;13 Suppl 3:S362–8.

43. Papavasilou AS. Management of the motor problems in cerebral palsy: a critical update for the clinician. Eur J Paediatri Neurol 2008; Sep 6 [Epub ahead of print].

44. Tilton AH. Management of spasticity in cerebral palsy. Semin Pediatr Neurol 2004;11(1):58–65.

45. Russman BS, Tilton AH, Gormley ME. Cerebral palsy: a rational approach to a treatment protocol and the role of botulinum toxin in treatment. Spasticity and other forms of muscle overactivity in the upper motor neuron syndrome. WE MOVE; p. 179–92. Available at: http://www.wemove.org. Accessed April 28, 2009.

46. Derstine JB, Shepard PM, Nixon-Cave K, et al. An interdisciplinary pediatric rehabilitation project I Vietnam: the Temple team experience. Rehabil Nurs 2003 May-June;28(3):92–5.

47. Fedreizzi E. Functioning multidisciplinary care and referral center for cerebral palsy. Childs Nerv Syst 1995;11:21–2.

48. Deepak Sharan. Recent advances in management of cerebral palsy. Indian Journal of pediatrics 2005;72:969–73.

49. Gulmans J, Vollenbroek-Hutten MM, Van Gemert-Pijnen JE, et al. Evaluating quality of patient care communication in integrated care settings: a mixed method approach. Int J Qual Health Care 2007;19(5):281–8.

50. Schwartz MH, Viehweger E, Stout J, et al. Comprehensive treatment of children with cerebral palsy: an outcome assessment. J Pediatr Orthop 2004;24(1):45–53.

51. Rémy-Néris O, Tiffreau V, Bouilland S, et al. Intrathecal baclofen in subjects with spastic hemiplegia: assessment of the antispastic effect during gait. Arch Phys Med Rehabil 2003 May;84(5):643–50.

52. Oefflinger D, Bagley A, Rogers S, et al. Outcome tools used for ambulatory children with cerebral palsy: responsiveness and minimum clinically important differences. Dev Med Child Neurol 2008;50:918–25.

53. Gracies JM, Elovic E, McGuire JR, et al. Traditional pharmacologic treatment for spasticity part I: local treatments. Spasticity and Other Forms of Muscle Overactivity in the Upper Motor Neuron Syndrome. WE MOVE self study guide. p. 57–78. Available at: http://www.wemove.org. Accessed April 28, 2009.

54. Gracies JM, Elovic E, McGuire JR, et al. Traditional pharmacologic treatment for spasticity Part II. Systemic treatment: spasticity and other forms of muscle overactivity in the upper motor neuron syndrome. WE MOVE self study guide. p. 79–110. Available at: http://www.wemove.org. Accessed April 28, 2009.

55. Tilton AH. Therapeutic intervention for tone abnormalities in cerebral palsy. NeuroRX 2006;3(2):1–8.
56. Steinbok P. Selection of treatment modalities in children with spastic cerebral palsy. Neurosurg Focus 2006, Aug 15;21(2):e4.1–8.
57. Mayer NH, Elovic EP. Neurotoxin Institute, practical aspects of botulinum neuro-toxin treatment of UMNS. Available at: http://www.NTI.org. Accessed April 28, 2009.
58. Albright AL. Intrathecal baclofen in cerebral palsy and movement disorders [review]. J Child Neurol 1996;11:S29–35.
59. Bottos M, Benedetti MG, Salucci P, et al. Botulinum toxin with and without casting in ambulant children with spastic diplegia: a clinical and functional assessment. Dev Med Child Neurol 2003;45(11):758–62.
60. Criswell SR, Crowner BE, Racette BA. The use of botulinum toxin therapy for lower extremity spasticity children with cerebral palsy. Neurosurg Focus 2006 Aug 15;21(2):e1.1–7.
61. Gooch JL, Patton CP. Combining botulinum toxin and phenol to manage spasticity in children. Arch Phys Med Rehabil 2004;85(7):1121–4.
62. Koman LA, Paterson Smith B, Balkrishnan R. Spasticity associated with cerebral palsy in children: guidelines for the use of botulinum toxin A. Paediatr Drugs 2003;5(1):11–23.
63. Scholtes VA, Dallmeijer AJ, Becher JG. Can we identify predictors of multilevel botulinum toxin A injections in children with cerebral palsy who walk with a flexed knee pattern? J Child Neurol 2008;23:628–34.
64. Tilton AH. Injectable neuromuscular blockade in the treatment of spasticity and movement disorders. J Child Neurol 2003;18:S50–66.
65. Berweck S, Schroeder AS, Gietzek UM, et al. Sonography-guided injection of botulinum toxin A in children with cerebral palsy. Neuropediatrics 2002;33:221–3.
66. Berweck S, Schroeder AS, Fietzek UM, et al. Sonography-guided injection of botulinum toxin in children with cerebral palsy. Lancet 2004;363(9404):249–50.
67. Willenborg MJ, Shilt JS, Smith BP, et al. Technique for iliopsoas ultrasound-guided active electromyography-directed botulinum A toxin injection in cerebral palsy. J Pediatr Orthop 2002;22(2):165–8.
68. Westhoff B, Seller K, Wild A, et al. Ultrasound-guided botulinum toxin injection technique for the iliopsoas muscle. Dev Med Child Neurol 2003;45(12):829–32.
69. Hägglund F, Andersson S, Düppe J, et al. Prevention of severe contractures might replace multilevel surgery in cerebral palsy: results of a population-based health care programme and new techniques to reduce spasticity. J Pediatr Orthop B 2005;14:269–73.
70. Novachek TF, Gage JR. Orthopedic management of spasticity in cerebral palsy. Childs Nerv Syst 2007;23(9):1015–31.
71. Barwood S, Baillieu C, Boyd R, et al. Analgesic effects of botulinum toxin A: a randomized, placebo-controlled clinical trial. Dev Med Child Neurol 2000;42(2):116–21.
72. Albright AL. Selective dorsal rhizotomy and the challenge of monitoring its long-term sequelae. J Neurosurg Pediatr 2008;1(3):178 [discussion: 178–9].
73. Bleyenheuft C, Filipetti P, Caldas C, et al. Experience with external pump trial prior to implantation for ITB in ambulatory patients with spastic cerebral palsy. Neurophysiol Clin 2007;37(1):23–8.
74. Gerszten PC, Albright AL, Barry MJ. Effect on ambulation of continuous intrathecal baclofen infusion. Pediatr Neurosurg 1997;27(1):40–4.

75. Langerak NG, Lamberts RP, Fieggen AG, et al. A prospective gait analysis study in patients with diplegic cerebral palsy 20 years after selective dorsal rhizotomy. J Neurosurg Pediatr 2008;1(3):180–6.
76. Sgouros S. Surgical management of spasticity of cerebral origin in children. Acta Neurochir Suppl 2007;97(part 1):193–203.
77. Abel MF, Damiano DL, Gilgannon M, et al. Biomechanical changes in gait following selective dorsal rhizotomy 2005;102(Suppl 2):157–62.
78. Gracies JM, Nance P, Elovic E, et al. Traditional pharmacological treatments for spasticity Part. Muscle Nerve Suppl 1997;6:S92–120 [review].
79. Gracies JM, Elovic E, McGuire J, et al. Traditional pharmacological treatments for spasticity part I. Muscle Nerve Suppl 1997;6:S61–91 [review].
80. Gracies JM, Simpson DM. Spastic Dystonia: etiology, clinical features, and treatment. WE MOVE; 2004. p. 195–211. Available at: http://www.wemove.org. Accessed April 28, 2009.
81. Gracies JM. Physiology of spastic paresis. II: Emergence of muscle overactivity. Muscle Nerve 2005;31(5):552–71 [review].
82. Brin MF, Comella CL. Pathophysiology of dystonia. Dystonia: Etiology, clinical features, and treatment. WE MOVE; 2004. p. 3–10. Available at: http://www. wemove.org. Accessed April 28, 2009.
83. Holton JL, Schneider SA, Ganesharan P, et al. Neuropathology of primary adult-onset dystonia. Neurology 2008 (Feb);70:695–9.
84. Banks HH. Equinus and cerebral palsy–its management. Foot Ankle 1983;4:149.
85. Barnett HE. Orthopedic surgery in cerebral palsy. J Am Med Assoc 1952;150:1396.
86. Graham HK, Baker R, Dobson F, et al. Multilevel orthopaedic surgery in group IV spastic hemiplegia. J Bone Joint Surg Br 2005;87:548.
87. Graham HK, Harvey A. Assessment of mobility after multi-level surgery for cerebral palsy. J Bone Joint Surg Br 2007;89:993.
88. DeLuca PA. The musculoskeletal management of children with cerebral palsy. Pediatr Clin North Am 1996;43:1135.
89. Renshaw TS, Green NE, Griffin PP, et al. Cerebral palsy: orthopaedic management. Instr Course Lect 1996;45:475.
90. Hagglund G, Lauge-Pedersen H, Wagner P. Characteristics of children with hip displacement in cerebral palsy. BMC Musculoskelet Disord 2007;8:101.
91. Abel MF, Damiano DL, Pannunzio M, et al. Muscle-tendon surgery in diplegic cerebral palsy: functional and mechanical changes. J Pediatr Orthop 1999;19: 366.
92. Boyd R, Graham HK. Botulinum toxin A in the management of children with cerebral palsy: indications and outcome. Eur J Neurol 1997;4(Suppl 2):S15.
93. Arnold AS, Anderson FC, Pandy MG, et al. Muscular contributions to hip and knee extension during the single limb stance phase of normal gait: a framework for investigating the causes of crouch gait. J Biomech 2005;38:2181.
94. Delp SL, Hess WE, Hungerford DS, et al. Variation of rotation moment arms with hip flexion. J Biomech 1999;32:493.
95. Hicks JL, Schwartz MH, Arnold AS, et al. Crouched postures reduce the capacity of muscles to extend the hip and knee during the single-limb stance phase of gait. J Biomech 2008;41:960.
96. Canale ST, Beaty JH. Operative pediatric orthopedics. 2nd edition. Mosby-Year Book; 1991. p. 664.
97. Chang WN, Tsirikos AI, Miller F, et al. Distal hamstring lengthening in ambulatory children with cerebral palsy: primary versus revision procedures. Gait Posture 2004;19:298.

98. Seniorou M, Thompson N, Harrington M, et al. Recovery of muscle strength following multi-level orthopaedic surgery in diplegic cerebral palsy. Gait Posture 2007;26:475.

99. Wolf TM, Clinkscales CM, Hamlin C. Flexor carpi ulnaris tendon transfers in cerebral palsy. J Hand Surg [Br] 1998;23:340.

100. Carlson MG, Athwal GS, Bueno RA. Treatment of the wrist and hand in cerebral palsy. J Hand Surg [Am] 2006;31:483.

101. Rayan GM, Young BT. Arthrodesis of the spastic wrist. J Hand Surg [Am] 1999; 24:944.

102. Sutherland DH, Santi M, Abel MF. Treatment of stiff-knee gait in cerebral palsy: a comparison by gait analysis of distal rectus femoris transfer versus proximal rectus release. J Pediatr Orthop 1990;10:433.

103. Vogt JC. Split anterior tibial transfer for spastic equinovarus foot deformity: retrospective study of 73 operated feet. J Foot Ankle Surg 1998;37:2.

104. Dodgin DA, De Swart RJ, Stefko RM, et al. Distal tibial/fibular derotation osteotomy for correction of tibial torsion: review of technique and results in 63 cases. J Pediatr Orthop 1998;18:95.

105. Gage J, Novacheck T. An update on the treatment of gait problems in cerebral palsy. J Pediatr Orthop B 2001;10:265.

106. Kay RM, Rethlefsen SA, Hale JM, et al. Comparison of proximal and distal rotational femoral osteotomy in children with cerebral palsy. J Pediatr Orthop 2003; 23:150.

107. Song HR, Carroll NC. Femoral varus derotation osteotomy with or without acetabuloplasty for unstable hips in cerebral palsy. J Pediatr Orthop 1998;18:62.

108. Mubarak SJ, Valencia FG, Wenger DR. One-stage correction of the spastic dislocated hip. Use of pericapsular acetabuloplasty to improve coverage. J Bone Joint Surg Am 1992;74:1347.

109. McNerney NP, Mubarak SJ, Wenger DR. One-stage correction of the dysplastic hip in cerebral palsy with the San Diego acetabuloplasty: results and complications in 104 hips. J Pediatr Orthop 2000;20:93.

110. Graham HK. Painful hip dislocation in cerebral palsy. Lancet 2002;359:907.

111. Saraph V, Zwick EB, Zwick G, et al. Effect of derotation osteotomy of the femur on hip and pelvis rotations in hemiplegic and diplegic children. J Pediatr Orthop B 2002;11:159.

112. Davids JR, Mason TA, Danko A, et al. Surgical management of hallux valgus deformity in children with cerebral palsy. J Pediatr Orthop 2001;21:89.

113. Andreacchio A, Orellana CA, Miller F, et al. Lateral column lengthening for planovalgus foot deformity in ambulatory children with cerebral palsy. J Pediatr Orthop 2000;20:501–5.

114. Noritake K, Yoshihashi Y, Miyata T. Calcaneal lengthening for planovalgus foot deformity in children with spastic cerebral palsy. J Pediatr Orthop B 2005;14: 274.

115. Thomson JD, Banta JV. Scoliosis in cerebral palsy: an overview and recent results. J Pediatr Orthop B 2001;10:6.

Bone Density in Cerebral Palsy

Christine Murray Houlihan, MD*, Richard D. Stevenson, MD

KEYWORDS

- Osteoporosis • Bone density • Bone health
- Cerebral palsy • Disabilities

Osteoporosis is a skeletal disorder characterized by compromised bone strength predisposing a person to an increased risk of fracture.[1] Osteoporosis remains a major health problem worldwide, costing an estimated $13.8 billion in health care each year in the United States. Despite advances in treating osteoporosis in the elderly, no cure exists. Osteoporosis has its roots in childhood. Accrual of bone mass occurs throughout childhood and early adulthood, and peak bone mass is a key determinant of the lifetime risk of osteoporosis. Because the foundation for skeletal health is established so early in life, osteoporosis prevention begins by optimizing gains in bone mineral throughout childhood and adolescence.[2,3]

Osteoporosis evaluation and prevention is relevant to children with cerebral palsy (CP). CP is the most prevalent childhood condition associated with osteoporosis. Bone density is significantly decreased, and children with CP often sustain painful fractures with minimal trauma that impair their function and quality of life. Preventing or improving osteoporosis and maximizing bone accrual during critical stages of growth will minimize the future lifelong risks of fractures in children with CP. This article addresses the anatomy and structure of bone and bone metabolism, the clinical assessment of bone mass, the causes of osteoporosis and its evaluation and treatment in children with CP.

OSTEOPOROSIS
Diagnosis in Adults

The diagnosis of osteoporosis in adults is well defined and based exclusively on the assessment of bone mineral density (BMD). Bone density is reported as a T-score which is the number of standard deviations more than or less than the mean for a healthy 30-year-old Caucasian (nonrace adjusted database) adult of the same sex. The World Health Organization classifies normal bone density as a T-score of −1 or higher. Osteopenia is classified as a T-score between −2.5 and −1, and osteoporosis is a T-score less than or equal to −2.5. If a person has a fracture and

Department of Pediatrics, University of Virginia, 2270 Ivy Road, Charlottesville, VA 22903, USA
* Corresponding author.
E-mail address: ch9g@virginia.edu (C.M. Houlihan).

Phys Med Rehabil Clin N Am 20 (2009) 493–508
doi:10.1016/j.pmr.2009.04.004
1047-9651/09/$ – see front matter © 2009 Elsevier Inc. All rights reserved.

a T-score of less than −2.5, then they are considered to have severe osteoporosis. Fracture risk and treatment options have been well investigated and documented in adults. Every 1 standard deviation decrease in BMD is associated with a twofold increase in fracture risk.[4] However, comparable information is limited in children.

Osteoporosis in Children

The risk of fracture associated with low BMD, the evaluation of osteoporosis, and treatment options in children are less well defined. However, over the past decade there have been advances in the diagnosis and diagnostic classifications for osteoporosis in children. The International Society of Clinical Densitometry released a position statement defining the parameters for the diagnosis of osteoporosis in children in 2008. Unlike adult osteoporosis, the consensus was that osteoporosis in children should not be determined based on densitometric criteria alone. The diagnosis of osteoporosis requires a clinically significant fracture history and low bone mineral content or bone mineral density (ISCD Pediatric Position Statement, 2008). The current definition for osteoporosis in children includes a BMD Z-score less than −2.0 adjusted for age, gender, and body size plus a clinically significant history of fracture: (1) 2 upper extremity fractures, or (2) vertebral compression fracture, or (3) a single lower extremity fracture. The Z-score is the number of standard deviations the patient's BMD is more than or less than age-, sex-matched reference values.

BONE EMBRYOLOGY, ANATOMY, AND ARCHITECTURE

To begin to understand osteoporosis a basic understanding of bone embryology, anatomy, and architecture is needed. The musculoskeletal system is derived from embryonic mesoderm at the third week of gestation. Mesenchyme, a subtype of mesoderm, is responsible for bone, cartilage, muscle, tendon, and fibrous connective tissue formation. In the sixth week of gestation, the mesenchymal cells begin the process of ossification of long bones. By the seventh week the cells differentiate into cartilage-forming precursors of long bones. In the eighth week the mesenchymal cells differentiate into osteoblasts, osteoclasts, and chrondroclasts through the process of endochondral ossification. This process transforms cartilage into bone and continues throughout childhood.[5]

Composition and Structure of Bone

The skeleton of the developing embryo is primarily composed of either fibrous membranes or hyaline cartilage, which provide the medium for ossification. The process of ossification of flat bones such as the skull, ileum, mandible, and scapula occurs through intramembranous ossification, whereas the long bones such as the tibia, femur, and humerus are formed through endochondral ossification. Each long bone is comprised of 2 wider ends (epiphyses), a tubular middle (diaphysis), and the developing zone between the 2 (metaphysis). A layer of cartilage (growth plate) separates the epiphysis and metaphysis in growing bones. This area becomes calcified and remodeled with bone when growth is complete. The outer layer of the bone is comprised of a thick dense layer of calcified tissue known as cortical bone, which provides strength to the bone. Eighty-ninety percent of the volume of cortical bone is calcified. Toward the metaphysis and epiphysis, the cortex becomes thinner and the space is filled with thin calcified trabeculae known as trabecular or cancellous bone. Only 15% to 25% of trabecular bone is calcified. The bone marrow, blood vessels, and connective tissue make up most of the space. There are also 2 surfaces that the bone has with the surrounding soft tissues. The external surface is the periosteal surface and the internal surface is known as the endosteal surface. These are lined with osteogenic cells, which maintain bone formation and absorption.[5]

Bone Formation and Absorption

The rates of absorption and deposition are equal in nongrowing bones. This delicate balance keeps the total bone mass constant and serves an important role in maintaining the strength of bones. Bones will adjust their strength in proportion to the amount of stress placed on them. Bones thicken with heavy loads and change shape to provide the necessary support. Healthy load-bearing bones and their trabeculae have enough strength to carry a load without breaking suddenly or in fatigue.[6] The deposition and absorption of bone aligns with stress patterns. New bone matrix replaces old brittle bone. This balance is maintained through the work of osteoblasts and osteoclasts.

Function of Osteoblasts and Osteoclasts

Osteoblasts are found on the outer surface of bone and in bone cavities. Osteoblast activity occurs in approximately 4% of all living bones. There is continual activity with new bone always being formed.[5] At the same time that bone is being formed, bone is also continually being absorbed by osteoclasts. Osteoclasts are large multinucleated cells. They are active on less than 1% of bone surfaces at any one time. Absorption occurs when osteoclasts send out villus-like projections toward bone and secrete proteolytic enzymes, citric acid, and lactic acid, which dissolve the organic matrix of the bone and the bone salts. The fragments of bone salts and collagen are than digested by the osteoclasts. Osteoclasts tunnel out sections of bone. Once the osteoclasts complete the process, osteoblasts invade the tunneled out bone and begin to lay down new bone.[5] Normal bones can detect and repair small amounts of microdamage. In some bones this damage can exceed the threshold, escape repair, accumulate, and result in fracture.[6]

Frost describes a hypothesis of mechanical bone competence that depends on the interactions between a bone's strength and the magnitude and types of peak voluntary mechanical load on a load-bearing bone during typical activities. Diseased bone or failure to achieve mechanical bone competence can result in nontraumatic fractures in childhood.[6] This can be seen in children with CP.

MARKERS OF BONE METABOLISM
Osteogenic Growth Factors

Insulin-like growth factors (IGF) are polypeptides that are synthesized in multiple tissues including bone. These peptides enhance the function of mature osteoblasts, therefore increasing bone matrix synthesis. Insulin-like growth factors inhibit bone collagen degradation and increase collagen synthesis, which help to maintain the bone matrix and bone mass. Alkaline phosphatase is secreted by osteoblasts while actively depositing bone. This activates collagen fibers and causes the deposition of calcium salts. The blood level of alkaline phosphatase is a good indicator of bone formation.[7]

The Role of Calcium and Vitamin D

Vitamin D plays a critical role in the mineralization of bone. It is produced in the skin through exposure to sunlight. Vitamin D is biologically inert and must undergo 2 hydroxylations, first in the liver and then the kidneys to become active (**Fig. 1**). The biologically active form is 1,25-dihydroxyvitamin D [1,25(OH)$_2$D]. Its role is to maintain serum calcium in the normal range. It does this by increasing the absorption of calcium

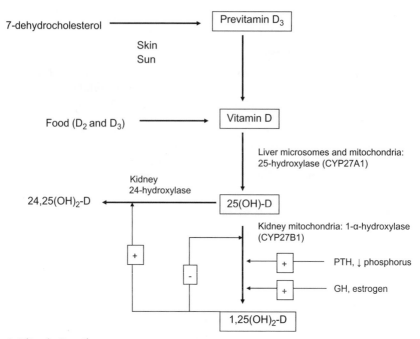

Fig. 1. Vitamin D pathway.

in the intestines and signaling stem cells in the bone to become mature osteoclasts. These osteoclasts then mobilize calcium from bone into circulation.[5] Vitamin D is found naturally in small amounts in some foods. Oily fish such as salmon, mackerel, and fish liver oils contain vitamin D. Bread products, cereals, milk, and other dairy products are fortified with vitamin D, although the percentage of fortification on the label may not accurately reflect what is found in the food.[8]

Vitamin D plays a role in bone mineralization by maintaining adequate levels of calcium and phosphorus in the blood. This allows the osteoblasts to lay down bone matrix. The production of 1,25(OH)$_2$D is regulated by serum calcium levels through the action of parathyroid hormone (PTH) and phosphorus. As vitamin D stores become depleted due to lack of sunlight exposure or dietary deficiency, intestinal absorption of calcium decreases from 30% to 40% to 10% to 15%. The decrease in calcium levels leads to an increased secretion of PTH. PTH signals the renal conversion of 25(OH)D to 1,25(OH)$_2$D indirectly through renal wasting of phosphorus resulting in decreased intracellular and blood levels. Hypophosphatemia in turn results in the increase in circulating concentrations of 1,25(OH)$_2$D. Multiple other hormones associated with growth and development (growth hormone [GH] and prolactin) also indirectly increase renal production of 1,25(OH)$_2$D.[5]

The 1,25(OH)$_2$D induces pre-osteoclasts to mature into osteoclasts. The osteoclasts in turn release hydrochloric acid and proteolytic enzymes that dissolve bone and matrix and release calcium into the extracellular space. 1,25(OH)$_2$D also increases the expression of alkaline phosphatase, osteocalcin, osteopontin, and cytokines in osteoblasts.[5]

FACTORS IMPACTING BONE MASS

Osteoporosis is a disease characterized by a reduction in bone mass accompanied by micro-architectural changes that reduce the bone's mechanical loading capability and increase its susceptibility to fractures.[9] Acquisition of BMD is multifactorial and includes nutritional factors, genetics, hormonal influences, and growth factors.[2] Gains in bone size and bone mineral content during childhood and adolescence are achieved only when environmental factors are favorable. Anorexia nervosa, exercise-induced amenorrhea, cystic fibrosis, inflammatory bowel disease, celiac disease, and rheumatologic disorders are associated with early deficits in bone mineral.[3]

Bone acquisition and remodeling is controlled by mechanical and metabolic factors. Normal skeletal growth, the progression of puberty, and bone mineral accrual all require appropriate hormonal influences, including thyroid hormone, GH, IGF, and sex steroids.[3,10] Bone growth is largely dependent on GH before puberty.[11] Later, sex steroids become essential for the completion of epiphyseal maturation and mineral accrual in adolescence. The importance of normal endocrine function for bone mineral accrual is highlighted by clinical deficiency states. Reduced bone mineral density is commonly seen in GH-deficient children,[12] and has been noted in disorders of estrogen resistance and aromatase deficiency.[13] Malnutrition, immobility, sex steroid deficiency, and other factors can interrupt bone mineral accrual and have been found to be a contributing factor to early bone loss in children with CP.[14]

Overall, appropriate gains in bone size and mineral content are achieved only when environmental conditions are favorable. Frost has discussed the idea that gene expression patterns in utero create baseline bone conditions at birth, including basic bony anatomy and anatomic relationships and neurologic and muscular anatomy and physiology. One also has the "machinery" to increase the strength of a load-bearing bone as needed by adapting to conditions placed on the bone during typical activities. However, factors that decrease a load-bearing bone's strength could potentiate non-traumatic fractures. According to the "mechanostat hypothesis," this could be the result of inadequate modeling, excessive disuse mode remodeling, impaired detection or repair of microdamage, degraded properties of bone that potentiate microdamage or a combination of the these.[6]

Adolescence is typically a period of maximal bone accrual. Recent studies suggest that attainment of peak bone mass occurs at a younger age than was previously believed, with the average age closer to 18 to 25 years than 30 years.[15–17] Twenty-five percent of peak bone mass is acquired during the 2-year period surrounding peak height velocity and at least 90% is reached by age 18 years.[11] If the process of bone accrual is disrupted during this sensitive period, profound and lifelong osteopenia can result. The label "female athlete triad" refers to a syndrome of disordered eating, amenorrhea, and osteopenia seen in adolescent women who engage in intensive physical training.[18–20] Expanding clinical experience with this syndrome confirms that the consequences of early osteopenia can be devastating. Premature fractures can occur, and lost bone mineral density may never be regained.[21] The characteristics of affected athletes may be analogous to those of pubertal children with CP, in whom impaired oral intake results in undernutrition and suboptimal body weight, delayed menses, and pubertal progression. This suggests a disruption of the hypothalamic–pituitary–gonadal (HPG) axis and abnormal hormone status.[22]

ASSESSMENT OF BONE HEALTH

The assessment of bone density is important for 3 reasons: to diagnose osteoporosis, to predict future fracture risk, and to monitor therapy.

Assessment of Bone Density Using Dual Radiograph Absorptiometry

Dual radiograph absorptiometry (DXA) is the most widely used method for assessment of BMD and is considered the "gold standard". DXA uses 2 different radiographic energies to record attenuation profiles at 2 different photon energies. Attenuation is largely determined by tissue density and thickness. At a low energy, bone attenuation is greater than soft tissue attenuation. At high energy, they are similar. This allows the distinction between bone and soft tissue. The energy absorption of the 2 different energy radiographic beams is used to provide estimates of the amounts of bone mineral. The radiographic photons are collimated into a fan beam that passes through the patients and the photons are selectively attenuated by the bone and soft tissue. After the beam passes through the patient, it is passed to a radiographic detector whereby the intensity of radiation is recorded. This provides a 2-dimensional measurement dependent on the size of the bone and does not separate cortical and trabecular BMD. It can measure central skeletal sites (hip and spine). Extensive epidemiologic data in adults have shown correlations with bone strength in vitro. The DXA scan has been validated in adults and is widely available in the United States (**Fig. 2**).

Bone density measured by DXA is an areal density (g/cm^2) rather than a volumetric density (g/cm^3). The BMD is the bone mineral content (in grams) per unit area (cm^2). The DXA scans are analyzed to generate measures of projected bone area, bone mineral content, and areal bone mineral density. Results are reported as T-scores in adults. This compares the patient's BMD with the young-normal mean BMD and expresses the difference as a standard deviation score. In children a Z-score is used. This compares BMD with age- and gender-matched references. Typical scan times for cooperative children are roughly 1 minute per scan for lumbar spine or distal femur and 5 to 7 minutes for the whole body.

In normal individuals, much of the pubertal gain in bone density as measured by DXA can be accounted for by increasing bone size. Increases in long bone diameter are matched by proportionate increases in cortical thickness, with no net increase in volumetric density.[23] However, bone strength is determined not only by bone density but also by bone geometry (eg, size of bone). Areal BMD may be diminished compared with age-matched normal subjects because of a true decrease in volumetric density or due to differences in the 3-dimenional structure of the bone.[24–27] Thinning of the cortex and a smaller outer diameter will both result in diminished areal density as measured by DXA, regardless of whether true volumetric density is decreased. The diameter of a cylindrical bone and the thickness of the cortex are important mechanical parameters. They have a significant impact on the ability of

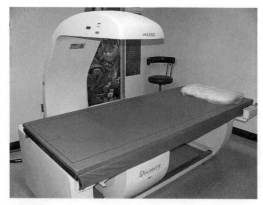

Fig. 2. DXA scanning device.

a bone to withstand loads without fracture.[27] Assessment of these factors is necessary to understand fracture risk, including in CP.

Assessment of Bone Density Using Peripheral Quantitative Computed Tomography

Peripheral quantitative computed tomography (pQCT) (**Fig. 3**) provides a 3-dimensional assessment of volumetric BMD. This differs from a DXA scan, which measures a 2-dimensional areal BMD. The limitations of DXA are relevant to growing children, as a DXA scan may not accurately capture changes in bone size that relate to bone strength. DXA can underestimate true volumetric BMD in growing children with small bone size. The advantages of pQCT are that it requires less radiation exposure and has good precision. The pQCT provides measures of bone size and geometry that are not attainable with DXA. The pQCT technology allows a 3-dimensional approach to measure bone density and bone geometry. This provides a more accurate assessment of change during growth. The pQCT is able to estimate cortical width and bone endosteal and periosteal circumference, allowing for better characterization of bone strength. Peripheral QCT is independent of size. Children with CP typically have smaller than normal bones with thin cortex. These are important parameters that impact on the bone's ability to withstand load and resistance to bending without fracture.[28] The use of pQCT is not yet widely used or validated in children with CP.

In addition, pQCT can distinguish between the 2 main types or compartments of bone: trabecular (eg, spine or distal radius) and cortical bone (eg, radial shaft). Trabecular and cortical bone differ in their rates of bone turnover and pattern of bone accrual during normal growth. Trabecular bone in particular is often more rapidly affected by disease or therapies. Peripheral QCT imaging obtains trabecular bone measurements at an ultradistal site, whereas cortical bone measurements are acquired from the shaft of the bone. The separate analysis of cortical and trabecular bone is also

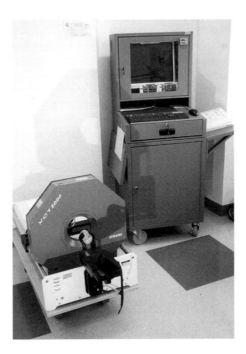

Fig. 3. pQCT device.

advantageous when studying the response to therapeutic interventions.[29] Measurements can include a potential weight-bearing site (tibia) and a non–weight-bearing site (radius). The trabecular site is evaluated at 4% of the length of the tibia or forearm. In addition, a second site at 20% of the length of the tibia or forearm is measured to assess a purely cortical bone. Bone mineral content, volumetric BMD, and area of the trabecular and cortical compartments can be calculated at both sites. Periosteal and endosteal circumferences and measurements of bone strength, the polar strength–strain index (pSSI), are measured at the 20% site. The pSSI is calculated considering the geometric properties (bone size) and material properties (bone density) of the bone. Settings to obtain the scans and analysis modes, including pSSI, in children with CP have been previously reported.[28] The scan time is approximately 90 seconds per slice (approximately 10 minutes total time).

Risks

Bone density scans (DXA and pQCT) expose the patient to a small amount of radiation. The total amount of radiation in performing DXA and pQCT (5 tests in total) is less than 4.0 mrem. The total radiation dose is similar to a round-trip cross-country plane flight, which is from 2 to 5 mrem per flight. The average background radiation to the general public is approximately 360 mrem per year. The total radiation exposure to complete these studies is therefore equivalent to a round-trip cross-country plane flight and is a small fraction (<2%) of the average background radiation that the general public receives per year. The risk from such a diagnostic procedure is not precisely known, but is believed to be small.

Challenges in Bone Density Assessment in CP

Assessment of bone density in children with CP has presented some challenges. Henderson and colleagues have been studying bone density and related factors in children with developmental disabilities including CP since 1993.[27,30–33] Henderson and colleagues[30] have demonstrated that reliable DXA measurements of bone density in children with CP may be obtained at the distal femur.[34] Assessment of bone mineral density in this region is clinically useful because this is the most common site of fractures. This innovative technique allows use of DXA technology in children whose spasticity or contractures preclude measurement at the traditional proximal femur site. Henderson and colleagues[26,27,30] have also compiled a database of DXA measurements (including distal femur values) in normal children, allowing standardization and comparison of DXA studies. Values for the reliability and coefficient of variation of the techniques are reported in these studies.

Peripheral QCT is not distorted by bone size or body weight, which is important when evaluating children with CP who often have smaller height and weight compared with age-matched peers. However, the assessment of bone density and strength in children with CP by pQCT also presents technical challenges. Binkley and colleagues[28] attempted pQCT scans in 15 children with moderate to severe CP. They were unable to obtain scans in 2 children due to issues with positioning in the scanner. They report on how to provide support for the extremities in children with CP, including splints to support legs, rolled towels, allowing the child to remain in their wheelchair, and help of staff to hold the necessary position.[28]

CP AND BONE HEALTH

Cerebral palsy is the most common physical disability of childhood.[35] Cerebral palsy describes a group of permanent disorders of the development of movement and posture, causing activity limitations, which are attributed to nonprogressive distur-bances that occurred in the developing fetal or infant brain. The motor disorders of cerebral palsy are often accompanied by disturbances of sensation, cognition, communication and behavior, epilepsy, and secondary musculoskeletal problems.[36] The average cumulative incidence rate of CP is 2.7 per 1000 live births. In recent years, the incidence rate of CP has been increasing internationally due to increased survival of low birth weight infants.[37–39] It has been estimated that more than 100,000 children in the United States today have some degree of neurologic disability attributed to CP.[40] Children with CP frequently grow slowly. The impact of this altered growth on skeletal development and bone density is a significant health problem. In typically growing children, the accrual of peak bone mass follows peak height velocity. However, in children with CP, differences in linear growth become more accentuated over time compared with their typically growing peers. In addition, as growth slows, the bone mineral density also falls further outside the normal range.

Growth in CP: Risk Factors for the Development of Osteoporosis

Bone growth, as assessed by BMD, is an important aspect of growth in children with CP. In addition to diminished linear growth, children with CP often sustain painful path-ologic fractures due to poor mineralization of bone, often with minimal trauma.[41,42] Thus, bone growth and bone density are highly relevant to overall linear growth, nutri-tional health, and health-related quality of life. Henderson and colleagues[30] initially investigated nutritional status and BMD in 139 children with CP in a cross-sectional study. They found that BMD was variable, but averaged −1SD. Functional severity (increasing severity) and lower nutritional status correlated with lower BMD. Low calcium intake and immobilization were also contributors to low BMD. Vitamin D levels and anticonvulsants did not correlate with BMD when the severity of CP and nutritional status were controlled. Serum calcium, alkaline phosphatase, and osteocalcin were also found not to correlate with BMD.

Henderson[31] then evaluated whether BMD can predict fractures in an observational cohort study of 43 children with quadriplegic CP followed for a mean of 3.8 years. During the follow-up, 9 fractures occurred. The predictive variables were history of a previous fracture and spica casting, but not lumbar spine BMD. Fractures in this population often occurred in the extremities or in the spine. Spine BMD did not corre-late well with BMD in the extremities, specifically the femur. However, in this popula-tion of children, who frequently have orthopedic surgeries, hardware, or contractures, assessment of BMD of the proximal femur could not be determined consistently. Subsequently, a new technique has been proposed for measuring BMD in the distal femur in children with CP in the lateral position, as this position can be more easily ob-tained in most children with CP and is more relevant to the site where fractures frequently occur. Scanning the hip was instituted in adults as this is the location at which fractures occur, but the distal femur is the most common location of fractures in individuals with CP.[34]

Further investigation into bone density in children with CP focused on those with moderate to severe motor impairment[27] (Gross Motor Function Classification System, GMFCS, III to V[43]). Significantly decreased bone density is virtually universal in non-ambulatory children with moderate to severe CP after the age of 10 years; however, predicting which children will fracture is a challenge.[27] Studies have found that the percentage of children with CP with a history of fractures ranges from 12% to 26%.[27,44] Multiple predisposing factors for bone fragility in individuals with disabilities have been investigated, including weight-bearing activity, muscle mass, calcium and phosphate homeostasis, nutrition, and medication use, especially glucocorticoids and anticonvulsants (**Table 1**).[14] In children with CP, these risk factors seem to disrupt bone homeostasis and result in microdamage that in turn predisposes them to non-traumatic fractures. Henderson and colleagues[45,46] have studied longitudinal assessments over 2 years of bone density in children and adolescents with moderate to severe CP (GMFCS III to V), finding that lower BMD Z-scores at initial evaluation were associated with greater severity of CP (GMFCS level), feeding difficulty, and poorer growth and nutrition as judged by weight Z-scores. Large variability in changes in bone density from +42% per year to −31% was seen in the distal femur and lumbar spine. Despite increases in BMD, distal femur BMD Z-scores decrease with age in this population.

Fracture rate was investigated by Stevenson and colleagues in a longitudinal cohort study of 245 patients with moderate to severe CP. At baseline, 15.7% reported a history of fractures. Children with fractures were older and had higher body fat content than those who did not fracture. Level of severity (GMFCS) and gender were not significant. Twenty children reported 24 fractures during 604 person-years of follow-up, with 4 fractures per 100 person years (4% per year). With a history of prior fracture at baseline, the rate increased to 7% per year. Having a gastrostomy tube (6.8% per year) and high body fat at baseline (9.7% per year) were also associated with increased risk of fracture.[47]

Binkley and colleagues[28] investigated bone density and strength assessment using pQCT in a cross-sectional study of 13 children with moderate to severe CP. Bone strength was compromised in children with CP secondary to smaller and thinner bones, not lower cortical bone density.

TREATMENT OPTIONS
Minimize Known Risk Factors

The first step in the management of osteoporosis in children with CP is to reduce the known risk factors. When possible, medications such as anticonvulsants that have the least impact on BMD should be chosen. Children need exposure to sunshine to maximize their absorption of vitamin D. Because sunscreen can reduce the ability to absorb vitamin D from the sun, 10 to 15 minutes of exposure 3 times a week before applying sunscreen are recommended.[5] The time needed can vary by location and time of year.

General Nutrition, Vitamin D and Calcium

Optimizing nutritional status, especially vitamin D and calcium levels, are important in the prevention and treatment of osteoporosis. Melanin reduces the production of vitamin D_3. Individuals with darker skin color require longer exposure (up to five- to tenfold) to sunlight to make the necessary vitamin D_3. Latitude, time of day, and season of the year affect the production of vitamin D_3 in the skin. Casual exposure

Table 1	
Risk factors for osteoporosis in CP	
Poor growth and nutritional status	Low calcium Intake
poor sun light	Immobility
Low vitamin D	Medications that interfere with vitamin D metabolism
Lack of weight bearing	Growth hormone insufficiency

to the sun provides most of the vitamin D needed. Excess is stored in fat to be used during winter months when exposure may be limited. However, topical use of sunscreen dramatically reduces the amount of vitamin D absorbed. A sun protection factor of 8 (SPF 8) reduces absorption by greater than 97%. Chronic sunscreen use can result in vitamin D deficiency.[5]

Vitamin D deficiency is a concern for children with CP who may not be exposed to ample amounts of sunshine and who may have insufficient dietary intake. Jekovec-Vrhovšek and colleagues evaluated BMD before and after supplementation with vitamin D and calcium. They followed 20 children with CP living in residential care. These children had severe motor impairment and used multiple and chronic anticonvulsant therapy. Thirteen children received vitamin D and 500 mg of calcium supplementation for 9 months. All children had increases in BMD. Of the 7 not treated and monitored, BMD remained the same or decreased.[48]

In 2008 the American Academy of Pediatrics (AAP) increased its recommendation for vitamin D supplementation for children. Exclusively and partially breastfed infants should receive supplements of 400 IU/d of vitamin D shortly after birth and continue supplementation until the child is weaned and consumes 1000 mL/d or more of vitamin D-fortified formula or whole milk. Nonbreastfed infants ingesting less than 1000 mL/d of vitamin D-fortified formula or milk should receive vitamin D supplementation of 400 IU/d. The AAP also recommends that children and adolescents who do not obtain 400 IU/d through vitamin D-fortified milk and foods should take a 400 IU vitamin D supplement daily.[49] The recommended daily intake of calcium varies based on age (**Table 2**).[50]

Vitamin D status can be determined by assessing levels of 25(OH)D. A level of less than 12.5 ng/mL is severe deficiency. Deficiency is defined as a level less than 37.5 ng/mL, and insufficiency as a level between 37.5 and 50 ng/mL. Sufficient levels of vitamin D are between 50 and 250 ng/mL. Aggressive therapy is needed for significant depletion. Pharmacologic doses of vitamin D should be used orally at 50,000 IU of vitamin D once weekly for 8 weeks.[5]

Activity and Weight Bearing

Caulton and colleagues[51] evaluated the impact of standing/weight bearing on BMD in a randomized clinical trial of 26 prepubertal children with severe CP, comparing children receiving 50% increase in regular standing versus no increase in standing for a 9-month period. Range of standing was between 180 and 675 minutes per week. Improvement in lumbar spine BMD of 6% was reported in the standing group over the control group. No change was seen in tibial BMD. These investigators concluded that, whereas increased standing may decrease the risk of vertebral fractures, it is

Table 2	
Recommended daily allowance of calcium intake	
Age	**Calcium Intake (mg/d)**
0–6 mo	210
7–12 mo	270
1–3 y	500
4–8 y	800
9–18 y	1300

unlikely to impact lower extremity fractures. The magnitude of an increase in BMD sufficient to decrease the risk of fracture has not been defined for children with CP.

Low Frequency Oscillation

Ward and colleagues[52] evaluated the influence of low-level mechanical stimulation on BMD in ambulatory children with disabilities in a double-blinded randomized control trial. Twenty children aged 4 to 19 years were randomized to standing on active or placebo devices for 10 minutes per day. Treatment was 5 days per week for 6 months. Volumetric trabecular BMD of the proximal tibia and spine (L_2) was assessed using 3-dimensional QCT. The children receiving low-level mechanical stimulation had improved BMD in the tibia after 6 months, compared with the children receiving sham treatment. This noninvasive, nonpharmacologic treatment option warrants further investigation in children with CP.

Growth Hormone

Administration of growth hormone (GH) has been shown to improve BMD in children with CP. Ali and colleagues[53] investigated GH treatment in a pilot randomized control study of 10 children with CP. Five children received GH daily for 18 doses. The remaining 5 children received no treatment. Linear growth improved significantly in the GH treatment group. Spinal BMD Z-scores, adjusted for height, also increased by 1.17 in the GH-treated group, in comparison to an increase of 0.24 ($P = .03$) in the control group.

Pharmacologic Bisphosphonates

Bisphosphonates are used to inhibit osteoclast-mediated bone resorption. In the United States, several bisphosphonates are available for use, including etidronate (Didronel), pamidronate (Aredia), alendronate (Fosamax), ibandronate (Boniva), and residronate (Actonel). Currently, none of the bisphosphonates are approved by the US Food and Drug Administration for use in children, and their use for osteoporosis in CP would be considered off-label in children.

Henderson and colleagues[54] investigated the use of pamidronate in a group of children with quadriplegic CP. Six pairs of children were matched within pairs for age, sex, and race. All the children had a BMD Z-score less than −2.0 and 11/12 had previous fractures. The treatment protocol involved a daily intravenous infusion for 3 days, with 3-day dosing repeated every 3 months for 1 year. The children were also followed for 6 months for observation after treatment ended. All children received calcium and vitamin D supplementation. Intravenous bisphosphonates safely and effectively increased BMD for the duration of the study. Although a promising treatment, for whom, when, and for how long bisphosphonate treatment should be considered remains uncertain. Although oral bisphosphonates are available, they have yet to be sufficiently studied in children, including those with CP. The impact on future fracture rates is unclear.

TAKE-HOME MESSAGE AND PLANS FOR THE FUTURE

Children with severe CP develop clinically significant osteopenia. Unlike elderly adults, this is not primarily from true losses in bone minerals, but from a rate of growth in bone mineral that is diminished relative to healthy children, a failure to accrue bone mass. The efficacy of interventions to increase BMD can only be assessed once the magnitude and natural course of bone maturation is understood in children with CP before

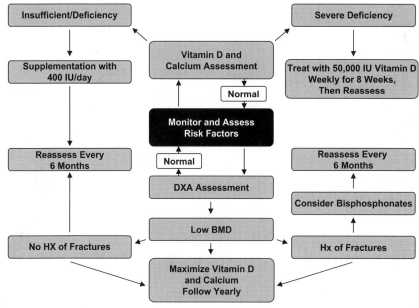

Fig. 4. Treatment algorithm.

intervention. There continues to be a need for research in the area of bone accrual, and prevention and treatment options for osteoporosis in children with CP.

Children with CP should have their risk of osteoporosis assessed at each visit. Calcium and vitamin D intake should be evaluated by the medical team. When necessary, supplementation should be started and levels followed closely. Available software for reference Z-scores for DXA scans for the lumbar spine begin at the age of 6 years. Reference Z-scores for the distal lateral femur are also available for children at the age of 6 years. If a child is considered at risk, DXA scans should be performed for a baseline at the age of 6 years with follow-up every 1 to 2 years depending on individual risk factors. If a child with CP meets the criteria for osteoporosis, the clinician also needs to consider the use of a bisphosphonate to improve BMD and possibly prevent future fractures (**Fig. 4**).

REFERENCES

1. NIH Consensus Development Panel on Osteoporosis Prevention, Diagnosis, and Therapy. Osteoporosis prevention, diagnosis, and therapy [see comment]. JAMA 2001;285:785–95.
2. Gelfand IM, DiMeglio LA. Bone mineral accrual and low bone mass: a pediatric perspective. Rev Endocr Metab Disord 2005;6(4):281–9.
3. Bachrach LK. Acquisition of optimal bone mass in childhood and adolescence. Trends Endocrinol Metab 2001;12(1):22–8.
4. Marshall D, Johnell O, Wedel H. Meta-analysis of how well measures of bone mineral density predict occurrence of osteoporotic fractures [see comment]. BMJ 1996;312(7041):1254–9.
5. Favus M, editor. Primer on the metabolic bone diseases and disorders of mineral metabolism. 5th edition. Washington, DC: The American Society for Bone and Mineral Research; 2003. p. 1–12, 129–37.

6. Frost HM. Bone's mechanostat: a 2003 update. Anat Rec A Discov Mol Cell Evol Biol 2003;275:1081–101.

7. Guyton A. Parathyroid hormone, calcitonin, calcium and phosphate metabolism, vitamin D, bone and teeth. In: Dreibelbis D, editor. Textbook of medical physiology. 2th edition. Philadelphia: Saunders Company; 1986. p. 937–53.

8. Holick MF. Photosynthesis, metabolism, and biologic actions of vitamin D. In: Glorieux JH, editor. Rickets. New York: Raven Press; 1991. p. 1–22.

9. Formica CA, Nieves JW, Cosman F, et al. Comparative assessment of bone mineral measurements using dual X-ray absorptiometry and peripheral quantitative computed tomography. Osteoporos Int 1998;8(5):460–7.

10. Bachrach LK. Bone mineralization in childhood and adolescence. Curr Opin Pediatr 1993;5(4):467–73.

11. Bailey DA, Martin AD, McKay HA, et al. Calcium accretion in girls and boys during puberty: a longitudinal analysis. J Bone Miner Res 2000;15(11): 2245–50.

12. Boot AM, Engels MA, Boerma GJ, et al. Changes in bone mineral density, body composition, and lipid metabolism during growth hormone (GH) treatment in children with GH deficiency. J Clin Endocrinol Metab 1997;82: 2423–8.

13. Carani C, Qin K, Simoni M, et al. Effect of testosterone and estradiol in a man with aromatase deficiency. N Engl J Med 1997;337(2):91–5.

14. Lloyd ME, Spector TD, Howard R. Osteoporosis in neurological disorders. J Neurol Neurosurg Psychiatr 2000;68(5):543–7.

15. Lu PW, Briody JN, Ogle GD, et al. Bone mineral density of total body, spine, and femoral neck in children and young adults: a cross-sectional and longitudinal study. J Bone Miner Res 1994;9(9):1451–8.

16. Matkovic V, Jelic T, Wardlaw GM, et al. Timing of peak bone mass in Caucasian females and its implication for the prevention of osteoporosis. Inference from a cross-sectional model. J Clin Invest 1994;93(2):799–808.

17. Vuori I. Peak bone mass and physical activity: a short review. Nutr Rev 1996; 54(4 Pt 2):S11–4.

18. Hobart JA, Smucker DR. The female athlete triad. Am Fam Physician 2000; 61(11):3357–64, 3367.

19. Sabatini S. The female athlete triad. Am J Med Sci 2001;322(4):193–5.

20. Skolnick AA. 'Female athlete triad' risk for women. JAMA 1993;270(8):921–3.

21. Drinkwater BL, Bruemner B, Chesnut CH III. Menstrual history as a determinant of current bone density in young athletes. JAMA 1990;263(4):545–8.

22. Hemingway C, McGrogan J, Freeman JM. Energy requirements of spasticity [see comment]. Dev Med Child Neurol 2001;43(4):277–8.

23. Seeman E. From density to structure: growing up and growing old on the surfaces of bone. J Bone Miner Res 1997;12(4):509–21.

24. Carter DR, Bouxsein ML, Marcus R. New approaches for interpreting projected bone densitometry data. J Bone Miner Res 1992;7(2):137–45.

25. Cowell CT, Lu PW, Lloyd-Jones SA, et al. Volumetric bone mineral density – a potential role in paediatrics. Acta Paediatr Suppl 1995;411:12–6 [discussion: 17].

26. Henderson RC, Lark RK, Newman JE, et al. Pediatric reference data for dual X-ray absorptiometric measures of normal bone density in the distal femur. AJR Am J Roentgenol 2002;178(2):439–43.

27. Henderson RC, Lark RK, Gurka MJ, et al. Bone density and metabolism in children and adolescents with moderate to severe cerebral palsy. Pediatrics 2002; 110:e5.

28. Binkley T, Johnson J, Vogel L, et al. Bone measurements by peripheral quantitative computed tomography (pQCT) in children with cerebral palsy. J Pediatr 2005;147:791–6.
29. Ward KA, Adams JE, Hangartner TN. Recommendations for thresholds for cortical bone geometry and density measurement by peripheral quantitative computed tomography. Calcif Tissue Int 2005;77(5):275–80.
30. Henderson RC, Lin PP, Greene WB. Bone-mineral density in children and adolescents who have spastic cerebral palsy. J Bone Joint Surg Am 1995;77:1671–81.
31. Henderson RC. Bone density and possible predictors of fracture risk in children and adolescents with spastic quadriplegia. Dev Med Child Neurol 1997;39: 224–7.
32. Henderson RC. The correlation between dual-energy X-ray absorptiometry measures of bone density in the proximal femur and lumbar spine of children. Skeletal Radiol 1997;26:544–7.
33. Lin PP, Henderson RC. Bone mineralization in the affected extremities of children with spastic hemiplegia. Dev Med Child Neurol 1996;38:782–6.
34. Harcke HT, Taylor A, Bachrach S, et al. Lateral femoral scan: an alternative method for assessing bone mineral density in children with cerebral palsy. Pediatr Radiol 1998;28:241–6.
35. Back S. Cerebral palsy. Philadelphia: WB Saunders; 1999.
36. Rosenbaum P, Paneth N, Leviton A, et al. A report: the definition and classification of cerebral palsy April 2006. Dev Med Child Neurol Suppl 2007;109:8–14.
37. Rosen MG, Dickinson JC. The incidence of cerebral palsy. Am J Obstet Gynecol 1992;167(2):417–23.
38. Suzuki J, Ito M. Incidence patterns of cerebral palsy in Shiga Prefecture, Japan, 1977–1991. Brain Dev 2002;24(1):39–48.
39. Colver AF, Gibson M, Hey EN, et al. Increasing rates of cerebral palsy across the severity spectrum in north-east England 1964–1993. The North of England Collaborative Cerebral Palsy Survey. Arch Dis Child Fetal Neonatal Ed 2000; 83(1):F7–12.
40. Kuban KC, Leviton A. Cerebral palsy. N Engl J Med 1994;330:188–95.
41. Bischof F, Basu D, Pettifor JM. Pathological long-bone fractures in residents with cerebral palsy in a long-term care facility in South Africa. Dev Med Child Neurol 2002;44:119–22.
42. Lohiya GS, Crinella FM, Tan-Figueroa L, et al. Fracture epidemiology and control in a developmental center. West J Med 1999;170(4):203–9.
43. Palisano R, Rosenbaum P, Walter S, et al. Development and reliability of a system to classify gross motor function in children with cerebral palsy. Dev Med Child Neurol 1997;39:214–23.
44. Leet AI, Mesfin A, Pichard C, et al. Fractures in children with cerebral palsy. J Pediatr Orthop 2006;26(5):624–7.
45. Henderson RC, Gilbert SR, Clement ME, et al. Altered skeletal maturation in moderate to severe cerebral palsy. Dev Med Child Neurol 2005;47:229–36.
46. Henderson RC, Kairalla JA, Barrington JW, et al. Longitudinal changes in bone density in children and adolescents with moderate to severe cerebral palsy. J Pediatr 2005;146:769–75.
47. Stevenson RD, Conaway M, Barrington JW, et al. Fracture rate in children with cerebral palsy. Pediatr Rehabil 2006;9:396–403.
48. Jekovec-Vrhovsek M, Kocijancic A, Prezelj J. Effect of vitamin D and calcium on bone mineral density in children with CP and epilepsy in full-time care. Dev Med Child Neurol 2000;42:403–5.

49. Wagner CL, Greer FR. Prevention of rickets and vitamin D deficiency in infants, children and adolescents. American Academy of Pediatrics Section on Breast-feeding, American Academy of Pediatrics Committee on Nutrition. Pediatrics 2008;122:1142–52.

50. Greer FR, Krebs NF, American Academy of Pediatrics Committee on Nutrition. Optimizing bone health and calcium intakes of infants, children, and adolescents. Pediatrics 2006;117:578–85.

51. Caulton JM, Ward KA, Alsop CW, et al. A randomized controlled trial of standing program on bone mineral density in non-ambulant children with cerebral palsy. Arch Dis Child 2004;89:131–5.

52. Ward K, Alsop C, Caulton J, et al. Low magnitude mechanical loading is osteo-genic in children with disabling conditions. J Bone Miner Res 2004;19:360–9.

53. Ali O, Shim M, Fowler E, et al. Growth hormone therapy improves bone mineral density in children with cerebral palsy: a preliminary pilot study. J Clin Endocrinol Metab 2007;92:932–7.

54. Henderson RC, Lark RK, Kecskemethy HH, et al. Bisphosphonates to treat osteo-penia in children with quadriplegic cerebral palsy: a randomized, placebo-controlled clinical trial. J Pediatr 2002;141:644–51.

The Adult with Cerebral Palsy: A Provider-Consumer Perspective

Kevin P. Murphy, MD[a],*, Kerstin Sobus, MD[b],
Patrick Michael Bliss, MA NACC.Cert[c]

KEYWORDS

• Cerebral palsy • Lifetime care • Adults

Advances in medical and surgical care over the past 20 years have resulted in children who formerly would have died at birth or in infancy now surviving into adulthood, many with significant, permanent physical disabilities,[1] including those due to cerebral palsy (CP). Increased awareness of these problems is needed by adult health care providers, who will be providing direct care to these individuals, and also by pediatric providers, who may be able to anticipate and prevent some of the long-term problems. The primary condition of CP, by definition, is non-progressive over time.[2–4] *Secondary conditions* are those that develop as a result of the primary condition and include entities such as soft tissue contractures, degenerative arthritis, and equinovalgus foot deformities. These conditions can be prevented with early diagnosis and appropriate intervention before problematic sequelae.[5,6] *Associated conditions* are those that occur with increased prevalence in individuals with CP, such as visual or auditory impairment, learning disability, and gastroesophageal reflux. These conditions are not necessarily preventable, but their impact may be lessened by early diagnosis and intervention during the developmental years. *Comorbid conditions* are those unrelated to the primary disability and appear with a similar frequency whether one has CP or not (eg, diabetes, hypertension). In the authors' experience, too often medical care providers blame the primary condition for just about all the symptoms and problems that can develop in the adult with CP. Symptoms such as leg pain, discomfort in the lower back region, and headaches are too often misattributed to the underlying condition of CP, giving no further pursuit to more specific and definitive diagnosis. For example, a person with CP presenting with a headache may be erroneously told

[a] Gillette Children's Specialty Healthcare, 1420 East London Road, Suite 210, Duluth, MN 55805, USA
[b] 1701 N. Senate Boulevard, Suite MT300, Indianapolis, IN 46202, USA
[c] Mercy Medical Center, Des Moines, IA 50314, USA
* Corresponding author.
E-mail address: kmurphy@gillettechildrens.com (K.P. Murphy).

Phys Med Rehabil Clin N Am 20 (2009) 509–522
doi:10.1016/j.pmr.2009.06.009
1047-9651/09/$ – see front matter © 2009 Elsevier Inc. All rights reserved.

that "all people with CP develop headaches at some point in time," with no additional diagnostics being offered. Strauss and colleagues[7] in reviewing the public health record for the State of California reported an up to 9 times higher risk of brain cancer in people with CP both young and old. As with any evaluation of an individual presenting with medical or surgical symptoms, the main initial goal should be to establish a correct diagnosis. This aim will be less frequently achieved if all loss of function and medical symptoms in individuals with CP are too easily attributed to the primary condition of CP.

Adults with CP, along with other individuals maturing with developmental conditions, are living longer, associated with improvements in medical and surgical care for all.[5,8–15] Estimates of the number of adults with CP in the United States have ranged between 400,000 and 500,000, depending on the defined age of an adult.[15] With aging comes an increase in the incidence of many conditions that can result in pain and significant loss of function over time. In addition to a possible higher risk of brain cancer in people with CP, Strauss and colleagues[7] also reported a 3 times higher risk of breast cancer and up to 4 times increased risk of cardiovascular death. Most of this higher risk is thought secondary to inadequate medical screening in the adult with CP. Inadequate screening in part relates to lack of education of the medical provider, undersized and inaccessible medical examination rooms and equipment, and not enough time being allotted to the provider for adequate history taking and physical evaluation. Communication barriers are especially significant for those adults who are nonverbal, require augmentative communication devices, or have expression of pain that is not recognized by the busy clinician. It is not uncommon to see adults with CP surviving well past 60 years of age and maintaining a functional lifestyle, with or without caregiver assistance.[16–19] Higher survival has been found in those adults with increased functional levels, ambulatory and with mat mobility, and in individuals with gastrostomy-tube feeding. Rimmer[20] was one of the first investigators to report that regular exercise improves functional status, decreases the level of required assistance, and reduces the incidence of secondary conditions in people with disability. Heller and colleagues[21] subsequently reported that exercise participation and frequency depended mostly on the care provider's attitude; if the care provider felt that exercise was important to the individual with physical disability, then exercise occurred.

A major premise in the care for the adult with CP is that major functional deterioration is almost always secondary to something other than the primary condition. Multiple diagnoses always need to be considered. It is not uncommon to have an adult with CP who also develops multiple sclerosis, Parkinson disease, Alzheimer disease, depression, cerebrovascular accident, or other associated or comorbid conditions. In the primary author's opinion, primitive reflexes, as well as a gradual trend toward more dystonia,[22] may be more noticeable with aging in this population.

ADULTS WITH CEREBRAL PALSY: COMMON MEDICAL-SURGICAL PROBLEMS AND THEIR MANAGEMENT
Spasticity

Spasticity persists beyond growth and development as a common threat to optimal function in the adult with CP. Botulinum toxin continues to have a significant role in management, relaxing hypertonic muscles for functional gain in the absence of fixed contractures. Botulinum toxin can be particularly helpful for those individuals with dystonia, either proximal or distal, in relieving painful spasms, improving vertical posture, and maximizing functional gain. Adults with CP may benefit from intrathecal baclofen, more commonly but not exclusively those of nonambulatory status. It is not uncommon to see catheter tip placements as high as the mid-cervical spine in individuals with more dystonia or upper extremity involvement.[22] Medical management of spasticity is addressed in further detail in the article by Damiano and colleagues in this issue. As noted by those investigators, most of the literature on the use of anti-spasticity medications in children is extrapolated from research on adult populations.

Orthopedic

Spine

Scoliosis can be present in up to 60% of adults with CP, and is particularly likely in those with nonambulatory status with spastic quadriparesis.[23] Progression with aging can occur at approximately 1° per year and should be monitored carefully over time. Progression can be accompanied by loss of function. Pain, when it occurs, is often associated with thoracolumbar soft tissue strain on the convex side and degenerative changes in facet joints on the concave side. Custom-molded seating or postural thoracolumbar orthoses can provide relief, along with other conservative measures such as episodic physical therapy and nonsteroidal anti-inflammatory drugs (NSAIDs). Scoliosis-related pain can be a new experience for the adult with CP, as scoliosis in children with CP is generally without pain.

Spondylolysis is thought to be an acquired condition related to a stress fracture through the pars interarticularis resulting from repetitive hyperextension.[24] The prevalence of spondylolysis has been estimated at 4.4% at 6 years of age, increasing to the adult rate of 6% at 14 years of age.[25] With one exception, a defect in the pars interarticularis has never been identified at birth.[26–29] Spondylolisthesis can be associated with spondylolysis, the development of which is felt to be infrequent after the age of 6 years in able-bodied children.[30] Reports in the literature have identified spondylolysis in weight-bearing adults with CP with an estimated prevalence between 21% and 30% in patients with or without dystonia.[31–33] The prevalence may be higher in individuals of status post selective posterior rhizotomy and with associated increased anterior pelvic tilt.[34–36] In a series of 143 patients who had never walked, in which the condition of CP was predominant, no case of spondylolysis or spondylolisthesis was detected radiographically.[37] Dystonic movements in the lumbosacral spine, particularly into extension and axial rotation, appear to be contributing to the higher incidence of spondylolysis in patients with CP.[32,38] It is not uncommon in the primary author's experience to see adults with CP having chronic back pain followed by their primary care providers for years. The back pain has usually been attributed to their primary condition of CP, believed to be expected and usual, and requiring no further diagnostic evaluation. Simple radiographs of the lumbar spine, including an oblique view, often reveal spondylolysis with low-grade spondylolisthesis, not uncommonly improving with basic conservative care. Symptoms typically improve within 6 months of treatment, including pelvic stabilization exercises, core strengthening, activity limitations, NSAIDs, and episodic use of a lumbosacral corset when helpful. Efforts to minimize significant anterior pelvic tilt in weight-bearing children may be helpful in preventing these potential stress fractures later in life, particularly in those undergoing selective posterior rhizotomy or aggressive hamstring lengthening, especially in the presence of tight hip flexor muscles.[39] Botulinum toxin injections into painful dystonic lumbar paraspinal muscles may be helpful in minimizing some of the extension and axial rotation that can contribute to future spondylolysis.[40] Gait aids and appropriate intermittent use of power mobility may provide additional protective factors. Careful monitoring through serial radiographs of the lumbar spine in those individuals with increased risk can allow early detection and intervention as appropriate. Surgical options including segmental fusion in the presence of failed conservative intervention, and any neurologic compromise should be used when necessary. Efforts to minimize toe walking should be provided, with use of appropriate orthoses when indicated. Symptomatic prestress fractures of the pars interarticularis also need to be considered and nuclear medicine bone scans may assist diagnosis. Medical history should include a review of any falls or injuries to the lumbar and pelvic regions, as more distant traumatic etiological factors may not be considered relevant by the individual at the time of medical evaluation.

Cervical stenosis has been found to occur with much higher incidence in adults with CP and athetosis than in normal controls.[41] Harada and colleagues studied 180 patients with CP and athetosis in comparison with 417 control subjects, and found an 8-fold increased frequency of early cervical disc degeneration and a 6- to 8-times increased frequency of listhetic instability in the mid-cervical spine in the individuals with athetoid CP. The combination of disc degeneration and listhetic instability with narrowed spinal canal was felt to predispose these individuals to rapid progressive loss of function and devastating neurologic deficit. Functional deterioration was also noted by Ando and Ueda[42] in approximately 35% of adults with CP, with a higher frequency among those with involuntary movements of the head and neck. Symptoms can include neck pain with loss of ambulation, progressive hypertonicity, and loss of bladder control and upper extremity function, occurring sometimes over a 6- to 18-month period. Additional studies focused on adults with CP and athetosis have associated higher incidence of cervical spondylosis and myelopathy, with dystonic head and neck postures.[43–51]

Serial magnetic resonance imaging scans every 2 years in individuals with higher risk, beginning in young adulthood, may facilitate early identification of cervical spondylosis and stenosis, allowing for more pro-active intervention and prevention of sequelae. Botulinum toxin injections may be helpful in minimizing cervical dystonia, particularly excessive movements into extension and axial rotation, along with improving posture and facilitating the fit of orthotic devices.[40] Medications for control of dystonia should be considered, including intrathecal baclofen therapy in carefully selected individuals. More calm environments and use of sensory biofeedback techniques and stress reduction strategies may also be helpful in reducing some regional dystonia. The primary author can recall a patient who, when flying alone in her glider plane, was completely relieved of all her dystonic symptoms until touchdown, when the ground support staff would come to her assistance. Cervical discomfort of any sort should be taken seriously in this population, as it may be the only prodrome recognizable before more devastating neurologic compromise. Serial neurologic examinations adapted for individuals with CP are also encouraged. Reproducible voluntary motor functions measured over time, along with a clinically reproducible spasticity measure, are suggested. Close monitoring of bowel and bladder functions for any changes, such as frequency, urgency, retention, and incontinence are not to be neglected. If conservative care fails, surgical decompression of the stenotic cervical canal may be required. A trend toward an anterior approach with interbody fusion and posterior wiring has been noted in the literature.[47,50,52–54] High risks of such surgery include regional dystonia postoperatively in the surgical zone, potential for aspiration, bleeding, and limited options for use of immobilization devices. Nonetheless, cervical stenosis associated with serious functional loss over time seems to be rapidly progressive in this population of patients with dystonic CP. Surgical intervention, despite the high risks, seems warranted when conservative care has failed to maintain function and comfort. Early identification and intervention should prevent potentially catastrophic sequelae of cervical stenosis in adults with CP and cervical dystonia, or at least minimize the surgical intervention required.

Hip

Hip displacement occurs in approximately 1% of patients with spastic hemiplegia, 5% with diplegia, and up to 55% in those with quadriplegia.[30,55] Pain with degenerative arthritis and joint space incongruity can occur in at least 50% of individuals with CP having dislocated hips or pseudo-acetabulum formation over time.[56–59] This problem is of particular concern in individuals having weight-bearing function in the lower extremities. Weight bearing can be limited, but important to the person functionally with standing pivot transfers, standing table usage on a regular basis, or during household or community ambulation or crawling. Pain and osteoarthritic changes can result in loss of functional weight bearing and mobility that is progressive over time. Early identification of hip dysplasia and intervention in the younger child should lead to prevention of significant hip subluxation/dislocation and pseudo-acetabulum formation in many individuals. Nonetheless, the painful arthritic hip, with or without dysplasia, in the adult with CP is not uncommon. Intra-articular injections with long-acting steroid and anesthetic can provide relief in the dysplastic, dislocated, or osteoarthritic hip for 6 months or longer. This procedure is often done under fluoroscopy, with previous arthrogram to identify needle placement, to assure optimal drug placement and disbursement throughout the painful bony interfaces. These injections can be combined with phenol injections to the obturator nerves to improve hip abduction and shift articulating surfaces to those with more cartilaginous cover. Periarticular botulinum toxin to address the painful adult hip can relieve additional tension myalgias and spasms, adding further relief. Total hip arthroplasties have been reported as safe and effective for selected individuals with CP having severe degenerative arthritis and pseudo-acetabulum formation.[31,60–62] Long-term follow-up studies have shown 94% pain relief and improved function over time even when operated on at a relatively young age of 30 years after hip arthroplasty.[63] Wear and tear seems to be minimal, which may relate to fewer steps per day and over time in the adult with CP. Proximal femoral resection-interposition arthroplasty may be helpful in individuals having no weight-bearing function in the lower extremities.[64,65] This is often a secondary procedure when more conservative care, such as intra-articular steroid, Botox, or phenol injections have not provided sufficient relief. The question of whether crawling is used for functional household mobility should be answered before surgical intervention, as most individuals will not offer this information on their own. The primary author has observed an individual of nonambulatory status but able to crawl within his home, with a painful dislocated osteoarthritic hip. This individual, having never been asked about crawling, had a proximal femoral resection performed at an outside institution. This operation eliminated his ability to crawl, resulting in the need to move out of his home and enter institutional care. The need to question adult individuals with CP regarding crawling behavior cannot be overemphasized. Self-injurious behavior must also be assessed pre- and postoperatively, as individuals can scratch their surgical incisions and disrupt traction units and immobilization devices if this problem is not carefully managed. Pain control needs to be carefully assessed, especially in those individuals with limited communication skills and variations of expression. Nonetheless, end-stage hip disease in functional weight-bearing adults with CP is virtually certain to result in loss of gait and mobility. In this scenario, total hip arthroplasties may be appropriate despite documented inherent risks and complications.

Knee

Patella alta is a relatively uncommon condition in ambulatory adults with CP, especially with spastic diplegia.[24,66] It is commonly associated with anterior knee pain in pre-adolescence or adolescence, with progression over time. An Insall ratio generally greater than 1 is observed on lateral radiographs.[67] The Insall ratio is determined by dividing the length of the patellar tendon (measured from the posterior surface of the lower pole of the patella to its insertion on top of the tibial tubercle) by the greatest diagonal length of the patella with the knee in 30° of flexion.[67] The ratio should be approximately 1 with less than 20% variation. The condition is commonly seen with crouch gait, limiting ambulation distance and contributing to further biomechanical and lever arm dysfunction on gait analysis.[39,68,69] Stress fractures may occur at the inferior pole of the patella, with palpable tenderness, requiring excision in the failure of conservative care.[31] Subluxations and dislocations of the patella are additional complications.[30,70]

Medical and surgical efforts to minimize crouch gait during the developmental and pre-adolescent years help prevent problems in adults with CP. These procedures include maximizing the knee-ankle-foot extension couple along with hamstring, quadriceps, and hip flexor stretching and strengthening muscles involved in weight bearing and gait.[34,71–73] Excessive tightness of the rectus femoris muscle, in particular, can contribute to the develop and persistence of patella alta.[31] In the primary author's opinion, more focus on quadriceps stretching in children with CP may be helpful in minimizing patella alta in adulthood. Increased prone-lying exercises and abdominal strengthening, minimizing anterior pelvic tilt, should additionally be beneficial. The young and middle-aged adult may benefit from patellar taping techniques to keep the patella more midline and tracking within the trochlear groove. Insall and colleagues[66] noted that clinical outcomes seemed to correlate more with patellar congruence than with severity of chondromalacia at the time of operation. Neoprene patellar tracking orthoses may provide additional reduction of symptoms in this regard. Intra-articular injections with a longer-acting steroid and anesthetic can provide more immediate relief, sometimes lasting 6 months or longer. The primary author has also used botulinum toxin A injections to the distal quadriceps mechanism, helping to relax somewhat the muscle adjacent to the superior patella. Injections are followed by a myofascial technique to lower the patella to a more inferior position closer to the center and midline of the knee joint. Physical therapy and NSAIDs can be of additional help as part of an overall conservative care program. With the failure of conservative care in the more skeletally mature individual with CP and progressive crouch gait, more aggressive surgical options should be considered. Such options can include multilevel operative interventions to correct femoral and tibial torsion, equinovalgus foot deformities along with distal femoral extension wedge osteotomies, patellar and tibial tubercle advancements, hamstring lengthening, and rectus femoris transfers.[39,69] Close monitoring of patella position over the developmental years, including a focus on preventative strategies as discussed earlier, may well prevent symptomatic patella alta later in life and the need for more aggressive multilevel orthopedic surgery.

Neurogenic Bladder

Neurogenic bladder does exist in CP and can be seen in up to 15% of the population.[74–82] It seems to be more common in those with bilateral involvement,[83] with an equal prevalence in males and females. Symptoms of frequency and urgency are most common, often associated with a hyperreflexic bladder of smaller volume. Anticholinergic medications can often relieve symptoms and provide continence in the absence of urinary retention. In the primary author's experience, the Mitrofanoff procedure (appendicovesical conduit), with or without bladder augmentation,[84] can provide continence and social confidence in carefully selected individuals with urinary retention, eliminating the need for indwelling catheters. For urinary retention secondary to detrusor sphincter dysynergia, the primary author has also successfully injected Botulinum toxin A into the pelvic floor musculature, relieving hypertonicity and outflow obstruction, sometimes repeated as an office procedure every 4 to 6 months. This procedure can facilitate urinary drainage in the absence of catheterizations. Upper tract pathology (hydronephrosis or vesicoureteral reflux) is rare in the adult with CP in the absence of urinary retention.[85–87] Medical providers should be asking more questions regarding bladder function in individuals with CP across the lifespan. This topic is often not raised by the patient, family, or other care providers, possibly secondary to a false assumption that urinary incontinence is just "part of living" with the primary condition of CP.

The conditions that have been discussed here are not uncommon in the adult with CP and should be anticipated by the specialty medical provider. Additional conditions specific to the adult with CP are becoming more recognized, but further discussion at this time is beyond the scope of this article. It is critical that the reader recognize that medical providers must not attribute every ache, pain, or loss of function presenting in the adult with CP to the primary condition of CP. Additional diagnostic inquiry is necessary as often secondary, associated, or comorbid conditions may be present and may be amenable to intervention. Practitioners focusing on children with CP need increased awareness of these problems in adults as interventions during childhood and adolescents may be helpful in prevention.

Identifying adult specialty providers and clinics can be difficult and resources vary geographically. There are few adult providers who have pursued training in conditions of childhood onset and few pediatric providers who are knowledgeable about the secondary, associated, or comorbid conditions manifesting in adulthood. Perhaps teaming of interested and capable pediatric and adult providers will facilitate the transition of youth with CP to adult providers. Networks and data banks of adult providers and clinics are being formed through organizations like the American Academy of Cerebral Palsy and Developmental Medicine and United Cerebral Palsy to help facilitate adult care and outcomes.

ACROSS THE LIFESPAN: AN INDIVIDUAL PERSPECTIVE

Cerebral palsy: I have investigated it, but even more I have lived it. I have felt its pain, tried to throw it away, deny it, felt its joy, known its promise, and felt its power. Over my 44 years, it has gone from my greatest anguish only to become my greatest strength and blessing. What a jump! Many will never understand this last statement, and it is not their responsibility. It is mine. I can tell you that my relationship with it is not perfect. We still have our moments. So far my life has been quite a journey—something I would never trade.

There are many ways to look at CP. It is important to understand that we who have CP have different views of it. Those families with individuals who have profound CP would look at its ramifications differently than those who have a family member with less severe CP. In addition, if I were to look at another person who has a mild case like I do, it still would not be the same or even equal. Why? Well, people are not only different physically; we are also different emotionally, psychologically, and spiritually. Our lives' journeys are diverse. CP encompasses our interactions with our "self" in reaction and interdependence to others. For example, when individuals get picked on or teased, while the words and actions used to cause the pain may be the same, the reaction is not. Pain and hurt affects the deepest part of us uniquely. I have heard the phrase "All human beings go through the same things." These words carry truth at a certain level, for all human beings share some basic degree of understanding, empathy, and compassion. Nonetheless, we need to be careful, because using these words without living in the shoes of the other can discount the person and what they may be experiencing.

By profession and vocation, I am a Chaplain for a hospital system. I have the privilege to work with children and parents. One of the areas I cover is the neonatal intensive care unit or NICU. I have met and work with parents who have been told that their little one has a high probability of having CP or another disability. The news of CP is devastating. First they blame themselves. I have heard, "What did we do wrong; is God punishing us, and what sin did we commit?" For mom and dad, at least at first, it can turn a child who is promising into a child who possesses unknown reality. Parents do not know what will happen next. What will be the extent of this disability? Will my child have other developmental issues? Will he or she go to school and will he or she even talk or walk? Is the condition mild or is it severe? Is this a livable situation or something that will crush my child, my family, and I? Can we rise above it?

Parents are the first who experience what a disability is and the pain of it. They need help to work through the emotion of it. They are most likely overwhelmed and will need help in processing the news and what it means. We must impart to parents, as they can consume, that life is not over but is still beginning. At this stage, it is important to have "compassionate distance." I define compassionate distance as being able to give love and empathy in one's practice without losing professional objectivity to provide the best medical care possible. Parents provide the foundation to the well-being and well-rounded growth of any child. This grounding is more important when a child with a disability is involved. Having a child with a disability can tear a relationship apart. I have seen it in my work as a chaplain. We may have to offer counseling. We need to show the parents that, while their child has this condition, he or she still has the promise and gift to be who they are. Parents will need help in developing coping skills and supportive relationships to walk this journey.

As the child enters school, he or she, for the first time, understands the phrase "I am different." This difference is not just in hair color, height, or weight. To the child it is the realization that I am "fundamentally different." I cannot speak; I cannot walk; I cannot be physical. I am different. Human beings, whether disabled or able-bodied, fear difference. We celebrate normal. Little ones with disability learn to hide by being quiet, playing alone. These children may not want to be noticed. This type of behavior can result in the creation of defense mechanisms. The child can grow and morph along ways of self-protection, leading him or her into an existence of being alone, including along the transition into adolescence and adulthood.

Parents are still providing the foundation. Parents cannot stop every pain, sadness, or hurt, but can provide something more powerful in the form of faith, hope, and love. If the parents take an avenue of "I will survive this," then the road may well be harder. This road can lead to overprotection, with the child not accepting his or her disability. Instead, the youth begins to see the disability as the enemy. There is a constant battle with the self that can lead to a damaged self image, shame, and self loathing, even following him or her into adulthood. From personal experience, I can tell you that CP cannot be conquered.

If the parents take the road of "we will thrive and be alive with this," so can the child, the adolescent, and the adult. Along this avenue, parents see the importance of not just accepting the condition of CP, but what I like to call "embracing it." As the person evolves from childhood to adolescence, he or she is beginning to understand CP as part of them. Through constant communication, support, and empowerment of family, friends, and professionals that help them, CP does not have to be fought or defeated.

CP can give one insights into life's meaning. CP can help one understand and help others, not in minor but in significant ways. CP can give "vision" into human nature, leading to greater compassion and understanding, possibly more than most have.

To say that adolescence is difficult is an understatement. We have the questions of: who am I, what is my purpose, and why? There is confusion, rebellion, hormones, relationships, and just trying to "figure it out." Now add a disability on top of that and what do you have? There is this constant want and need to fit and to be accepted, but it is hard to be accepted when others cannot accept themselves. One of the hardest things to teach teens is that there are some people who will never understand. It is not possible to get through the barrier that protects the hearts of some people. School remains the main arena for socialization. It is hard. The truth of the matter is that we learn who we are and how we fit mostly by going through adversity. We learn to cope and gain confidence mostly by walking through the pain. Therefore, as in childhood, we must watch for any behavior in adolescence that indicates withdrawal or isolation. Counseling may be appropriate with a religious leader or other professional. As with children, we must advocate for social activities, whether sports, choir, drama, or other school or healthy community pursuit. These activities will aid in learning to cope.

Pain can add up. Out of fear of reprisals, individuals with disabilities will not speak up. Emotions are swallowed. As with children, it is important that we form relationships that go beyond just caring for the CP. The whole person needs tending to—body, mind, and soul. It is imperative to ask how the individual's life is going. How is home, school, and other relationships? Asking these questions may help engender trust, speak to what is going on, and provide emotional comfort. This in turn can help the youth to grow in confidence, improving participation in therapy services, household duties, and other activities.

The teen years are all about individuality and sibling relationships are important. During this life period, one is still defined by where he or she came from, including whose mom, whose dad, and whose brother or sister is disabled. Siblings of one who has CP have to at times put up with teasing and ridicule, which may lead to resentment toward the individual with CP. Another issue in the family dynamics is the other siblings feeling that their brother or sister with CP is the favorite, the perfect one, or the one that gets most or all of the attention. We must be able to help families be a stronger unit, especially when a disability is involved. Families will need our assistance in learning how to share thoughts, feelings, joy, or pain. Communication, understanding, and love are the keys, with the family being the springboard to success.

College is freedom, but can be fearsome. This period is an important transition time for both the person with CP and the parents. Here is where all of the last 18 years of raising a child is tested. Letting go is hard for all parents, and even more so for those who have a child with a disability. "I can't protect him or her any more." "What if something happens?" College offers a new level of growth, with more self reliance. At this point we see the results of the choice of either "I will survive" or "I will thrive." It can be especially hard for a young person with CP to leave home, as he or she is leaving all that was comfortable and going into all that is unknown. Many colleges have ways to integrate students with disabilities and finding one more compatible with the young person's special needs can make all the difference.

Adulthood has come. All decisions are ours. Parents, while still important and needed, are given a new position of friend and advisor. Adulthood is also a time of more revealed truth. When one is a child and teen, he or she may believe that, once attaining college and adulthood, relationships will be far easier and there will be no teasing or even discrimination. This is not exactly true. A hope of mine that was shattered was that adults just know better; some do not. Professors still may stereotype intellects as "not great," lowering expectations as "this is all you can be expected to do." In addition, some professors may see struggling as a manifestation of not accepting limitations. Intellectual capacity is still too often seen as directly connected to physical capacity. Although learning disabilities can be (but are not necessarily) part of having CP, there is still capability to achieve. Navigating college might be facilitated by getting in touch with the disability services. Tutoring and other learning aids may be helpful, if needed.

Leaving school and entering the world of work introduces new challenges. A person with CP at this stage, as during childhood and in adolescence, can try too hard. The phrase "just be yourself" may still be "foggy." One comes to understand that integration can take a lifetime and that it is important to continue to work on this process. Counseling whenever needed can be helpful. Age and time teaches one to let go. It remains important to have a support team of family, friends, and professionals. Vocational rehabilitation offers programs to help individuals to find appropriate employment and keep engaged in the job market. It may take time to find one's niche; one may even go through one or more jobs. Using the support team that a person has, with or without CP, will help in this area.

As one transitions from adolescence to adulthood, it is important to keep going to one's doctor. Young adults should be encouraged strongly here, because the body does change. I have found that not all doctors are equal in this regard, so help should be given to find the right one. Why is it important to find the right doctor and other health care providers? Quite simply, there are professionals out there that see only the condition of CP and not the person. If we do not see the person, the condition will not improve, nor necessarily even remain stable, and the person will not heal in all aspects. There are some doctors and professionals who should not work with persons with CP or other disabilities, as they do not understand the holistic way that CP affects one's life. For these providers, the person with disability is not seen as a person to relate to, understand, or learn from, but a burden.

It is important that one stays engaged in friendship, family, church, and community organizations. Isolation is still possible as an adult, so any way that we can help those with CP or other disabilities to stay "other-focused" is wonderful. Professionals should be diligent in looking for signs of depression or isolation, as it may be that any past unresolved issue will arise. As I have found, if the past is not healed, it will dictate one's future. CP can be a glass through which one sees others, including relationships, work, and buying a house or a car. For example, when purchasing a house, issues include those of practicality and function; steps, yard, and anything that could affect the livability of the person with CP warrants investigation.

Relationships have come easier to me because I have grown and worked on my own issues. Point to be taken: it is not always them, it is sometimes us. For example, if one worries too much that rejection is around the corner, it may be. Relationships are core and need to be seen as such. That is why the support of friends, family, and professionals are so important. As with all individuals, we cannot be mirrors unto ourselves. We will need truthful support. Most of the time, for myself, it has not been the CP that has been the issue, but everything that revolves around it. Relationship is at the heart. I have found that we are meant to be relational, not islands.

The most important thing I have ever learned is that having CP is not the end. Living with it has not been easy, but there is no more denying. The grace it has given me has enabled me not to become bitter. I have discovered my greater purpose in having CP, as it helps me to help other people. If I can help another find purpose, love, meaning, and truth in this life, then having CP is worth it.

REFERENCES

1. Hallum A. Disability and the transition to adulthood: issues for the disabled child, the family, and the pediatrician. Curr Probl Pediatr 1995;25:12–50.
2. Ropper AH, Brown RH. Adams and Victor's principles of neurology. 8th edition. Columbus: McGraw-Hill Companies Inc.; 2005.
3. McCormick A, Brien M, Plourde J, et al. Stability of Gross Motor Function Classification System in adults with cerebral palsy. Dev Med Child Neurol 2007;49: 265–9.
4. Rosenbaum P, Paneth N, Leviton A, et al. A report: the definition and classification of cerebral palsy April 2006. Dev Med Child Neurol Suppl 2007;109: 8–14.
5. Turk MA, Scandale MS, Rosenbaum PF, et al. The health of women with cerebral palsy. Phys Med Rehabil Clin N Am 2001;12(1):153–68.
6. Turk MA, Geremski CA, Rosenbaum PF, et al. The health status of women with cerebral palsy. Arch Phys Med Rehabil 1997;78:10–7.
7. Strauss D, Cable W, Shavelle R. Causes of excess mortality in cerebral palsy. Dev Med Child Neurol 1999;41:580–5.
8. Murphy KP. Medical problems in adults with cerebral palsy: case examples. Assist Technol 1999;11:97–104.
9. Granet KM, Balaghi M, Jaeger J, et al. Adults with cerebral palsy. N J Med 1997; 94:51–4.
10. Murphy KP, Molnar GE, Lankasky K, et al. Medical and functional status of adults with cerebral palsy. Dev Med Child Neurol 1995;37:1075–84.
11. Murphy KP, Molnar GE, Lankasky K, et al. Employment and social issues in adults with cerebral palsy. Arch Phys Med Rehabil 2000;81:807–11.
12. Young NL, Steele C, Fehlings D, et al. Use of healthcare among adults with chronic and complex physical disabilities of childhood. Disabil Rehabil 2005; 27(23):1455–60.
13. Rimmer JH. Physical fitness levels of persons with cerebral palsy. Dev Med Child Neurol 2001;43:208–12.
14. Hemming K, Steele C, Fehlings D, et al. Long-term survival for a cohort of adults with cerebral palsy. Dev Med Child Neurol 2006;48:90–5.
15. Rapp CE, Torres MM. The adult with cerebral palsy. Arch Fam Med 2000;9: 466–72.
16. Strauss D, Shavelle R. Life expectancy of adults with cerebral palsy. Dev Med Child Neurol 1998;40:369–75.
17. Strauss E, Ojdana K, Shavelle R, et al. Decline in function and life expectancy of older persons with cerebral palsy. NeuroRehabilitation 2004;19:69–78.
18. Strauss D, Shavelle R, Reynolds R, et al. Survival in cerebral palsy in the last 20 years: signs of improvement? Dev Med Child Neurol 2007;49:86–92.
19. Strauss D, Brooks J, Rosenbloom L, et al. Life expectancy in cerebral palsy: an update. Dev Med Child Neurol 2008;50:487–93.
20. Rimmer JH. Health promotion for people with disabilities. Phys Ther 1999;79(5): 495–502.
21. Heller T, Ying Gui-shuang, Rimmer James H, et al. Determinants of exercise in adults with cerebral palsy. Public Health Nurs 2002;19(3):223–31.
22. Albright AL. Principles & practice of pediatric neurosurgery. 2nd edition. New York: Thieme Medical Publishers, Inc.; 2008.
23. Lonstein JE, Bradford DS, Winter RB, et al. Moe's textbook of scoliosis & other spine deformities. 3rd edition. Philadelphia: WB Saunders Company; 1995.

24. Able MF. Orthopedic knowledge update. Rosemont (IL): American Academy of Orthopedic Surgeons; 2006.
25. Fredrickson BE, Baker D, McHolick WJ, et al. The natural history of spondylolysis and spondylolisthesis. J Bone Joint Surg Am 1984;66:699–707.
26. Borkow SE, Kleiger B. Spondylolisthesis in the newborn. A case report. Clin Orthop Relat Res 1971;81:73–6.
27. Newnan PH. The etiology of spondylolisthesis. J Bone Joint Surg Br 1963;45:39–59.
28. Taillard WF. Etiology of spondylolisthesis. Clin Orthop Relat Res 1976;117:30–9.
29. Beguiristain JL, Diaz-de-Rada P. Spondylolisthesis in preschool children. J Pediatr Orthop B 2004;13:225–30.
30. Morrissy RT, Weinstein SL. Lovell and Winter's pediatric orthopedics. 6th edition. Philadelphia: Lippencott, Williams and Wilkins; 2006.
31. Morrell DS, et al. Progressive bone and joint abnormalities of the spine and lower extremities in cerebral palsy. Radiographics 2002;22:257–68.
32. Sakai T, Katoh S, SaSa T, et al. Lumbar spinal disorders in patients with athetoid cerebral palsy: a clinical and biomechanical study. Spine 2006;31(3):E66–70.
33. Harada T, Ebara S, Anwar MM, et al. Lumbar spine and patients with spastic diplegia. J Bone Joint Surg Br 1993;75:534–7.
34. Peter JC, Hoffman EB, Arens LJ, et al. Incidence of spinal deformity in children after multiple level laminectomy for selective posterior rhizotomy. Childs Nerv Syst 1990;6:30–2.
35. Li Z, Zhu J, Liu X, et al. Deformity of lumbar spine after selective dorsal rhizotomy for spastic cerebral palsy. Microsurgery 2008;28:10–2.
36. Peter JC, Hoffman EB, Arens LJ, et al. Spondylolysis and spondylolisthesis after five level lumbosacral laminectomy for selective posterior rhizotomy in cerebral palsy. Childs Nerv Syst 1993;9:285–8.
37. Rosenberg NJ, Bargar WL, Friedman B, et al. The incidence of spondylolysis and spondylolistheses in non-ambulatory patients. Spine 1981;6(1):35–8.
38. Wang JP, Shou-Yu C, Yates P, et al. Finite element analysis of the spondylolysis in lumbar spine. Biomed Mater Eng 2006;16:301–8.
39. Gage JR. The treatment of gait problems in cerebral palsy. Clinics in developmental medicine. London: Mac Keith Press; 2004. p.165.
40. Gallien P, Nicolas B, Petrilli S, et al. Role for botulinum toxin in back pain treatment in adults with cerebral palsy: report of a case. Joint Bone Spine 2004;71:76–8.
41. Harada T, Ebara S, Anwar MM, et al. The cervical spine in athetoid cerebral palsy, a radiologic study of 180 patients. J Bone Joint Surg Br 1996;78(4):613–9.
42. Ando N, Ueda S. Functional deterioration in adults with cerebral palsy. Clin Rehabil 2000;14:300–6.
43. Reese ME, Msall ME, Owen S, et al. Acquired cervical spine impairment in young adults with cerebral palsy. Dev Med Child Neurol 1991;33:153–66.
44. Anderson WW, Wise BL, Itabashi HH, et al. Cervical spondylosis in patients with athetosis. Neurology 1962;12:410–2.
45. Levine RA, Rosenbaum AE, Waltz JM, et al. Cervical spondylosis and dyskinesias. Neurology 1970;20:1194–9.
46. Angeline L, Broggi G, Nardocci M, et al. Subacute cervical myelopathy in a child with cerebral palsy. Secondary to torsion dystonia? Childs Brain 1982;9:354–7.
47. Fuji T, Yonenobu K, Fujiwara K, et al. Cervical radiculopathy or myelopathy secondary to athetoid cerebral palsy. J Bone Joint Surg Am 1987;69:815–21.
48. Nokura K, Hashizume Y, Inagaki T, et al. Clinical and pathological study of myelopathy accompanied with cervical spinal canal stenosis with special

reference to complication of mental retardation or cerebral palsy. Rinsho Shinkei-gaku 1993;33:121–9 [in Japanese].

49. Hrose G, Kadoya S. Cervical spondylitic radiculo-myelopathy in patients with athetoid-dystonic cerebral palsy: clinical evaluation and surgical treatment. J Neurol Neurosurg Psychiatry 1984;47:775–80.

50. Pollak L, Schiffer J, Klein C, et al. Neurosurgical intervention for cervical disc disease in dystonic cerebral palsy. Mov Disord 1998;13(4):713–7.

51. Ebara S, Harada T, Yamamoto Y, et al. Unstable cervical spine in athetoid cerebral palsy. Spine 1989;14:1154–9.

52. Nishihara N, Tanabe G, Nakahara S, et al. Surgical treatment of cervical spondylotic myelopathy complicating athetoid cerebral palsy. J Bone Joint Surg Br 1984; 66:504–8.

53. Bishop RS, Moore KA, Hadley MN, et al. Anterior cervical interbody fusion using autogenic and allogenic bone graft substrate. J Neurosurg 1996;85:206–10.

54. Connolly PJ, Esses SI, Kostuik JP, et al. Anterior cervical fusion outcome analysis of patients fused with and without anterior cervical plates. J Spinal Disord 1996;9: 202–6.

55. Laplaza FJ, Root L, Tassanawipas A, et al. Femoral torsion and neck shaft angles in cerebral palsy. J Pediatr Orthop 1993;13:192–9.

56. Cooperman DR, Bartucci E, Dietrick E, et al. Hip dislocations in spastic cerebral palsy: long-term consequences. J Pediatr Orthop 1987;7:268–76.

57. Moreau M, Drummond DS, Rogala E, et al. Natural history of the dislocated hip in spastic cerebral palsy. Dev Med Child Neurol 1979;21:749–53.

58. Pritchett JW. Treated and untreated unstable hips in severe cerebral palsy. Dev Med Child Neurol 1990;32:3–6.

59. Hodgkinson I, Jindrich ML, Duhaut P, et al. Hip pain in adults with cerebral palsy. Dev Med Child Neurol 2001;43:806–8.

60. Koffman M. Proximal femoral resection or total hip replacement in severely disabled cerebral spastic patients. Orthop Clin North Am 1981;12:91–100.

61. Root L, Spero CR. Hip adductor transfer compared with adductor tenotomy in cerebral palsy. J Bone Joint Surg Am 1981;63:767–72.

62. Root L, Goss JR, Mendes J. The treatment of the painful hip in cerebral palsy by total hip replacement or hip arthrodesis. J Bone Joint Surg Am 1986;68:590–8.

63. Buly RL, Huo M, Root L, et al. Total hip arthroplasty in cerebral palsy. Long-term follow-up results. Clin Orthop Relat Res 1993;296:148–53.

64. McCarthy RE, Douglas B, Zawacli RP, et al. Proximal femoral resection to allow adults who have severe cerebral palsy to sit. J Bone Joint Surg Am 1988;70: 1011–6.

65. Widmann RF, Do TT, Doyle SM, et al. Resection arthroplasty of the hip for patients with cerebral palsy: an outcome study. J Pediatr Orthop 1999;19:805–10.

66. Insall JN, Aglietti P, Tria AJ Jr. Patellar pain and incongruence, clinical application. Clin Orthop Relat Res 1983;176:225–32.

67. Aglietti P, Aglietti P, Tria AJ. Patellar pain and incongruence, measurements of incongruence. Clin Orthop Relat Res 1983;176:217–24.

68. Hoffinger SA, Rad GT, Abou-Ghaida H. Hamstrings in cerebral palsy crouched gait. J Pediatr Orthop 1993;13:722–6.

69. Rodda JM, Graham HK, Carson L, et al. Correction of severe crouched gait in patients with spastic diplegia with use of multilevel orthopedic surgery. J Bone Joint Surg Am 2006;88(12):2653–64.

70. Simmons E, Cameron JC. Patella alta and recurrent dislocation of the patella. Clin Orthop Relat Res 1992;274:265–9.

71. Andersson C, Grooten W, Hellsten M, et al. Adults with cerebral palsy: walking ability after progressive strength training. Dev Med Child Neurol 2003;45:220–8.
72. Taylor NF, Dodd KJ, Larkin H. Adults with cerebral palsy benefit from participating in a strength training program and a community gymnasium. Disabil Rehabil 2004;26(19):1128–34.
73. Allen J, Dodd KJ, Taylor NF, et al. Strength training can be enjoyable and beneficial for adults with cerebral palsy. Disabil Rehabil 2004;26(19):1121–7.
74. Sweetser PM, Badell A, Schneider S, et al. Effects of sacral dorsal rhizotomy on bladder function in patients with spastic cerebral palsy. Neurourol Urodyn 1995; 14:57–64.
75. Houle AM, Vernet O, Jednak R, et al. Bladder function before and after selective dorsal rhizotomy in children with cerebral palsy. J Urol 1998;160:1088–91.
76. Reid CJ, Borzyskowski M. Lower urinary tract dysfunction in cerebral palsy. Arch Dis Child 1993;68:739–42.
77. McNeal DM, Hawtrey CE, Wolraich ML, et al. Symptomatic neurogenic bladder in a cerebral palsied population. Dev Med Child Neurol 1983;5:612–6.
78. Decter RM, Bauer SB, Khoshbin S, et al. Urodynamic assessment of children with cerebral palsy. J Urol 1987;138:1110–2.
79. Drigo P, Seren F, Artibani W, et al. Neurogenic vesicourethral dysfunction in children with cerebral palsy. Ital J Neurol Sci 1988;9:151–4.
80. Karaman M, Kaya C, Caskurlu T, et al. Urodynamic findings in children with cerebral palsy. Int J Urol 2005;12:717–20.
81. Bross S, Pomer S, Doderlein L, et al. Urodynamic findings in patients with infantile cerebral palsy. Aktuelle Urol 2004;35:54–7 [in German].
82. Borzyskowski M. Cerebral palsy and the bladder. Dev Med Child Neurol 1989;31: 687–9.
83. Edby K, Marild S. Urinary tract dysfunction in children with cerebral palsy. Acta Paediatr 2000;12:1505–6.
84. Cain M, Rink EB, Yerkes M, et al. Appendicovesicostomy and newer alternatives for the Mitroffanoff procedure: results in the last 100 patients at Riley Children's Hospital. J Urol 1999;162(5):1749–52.
85. Mayo ME. Lower urinary tract dysfunction in cerebral palsy. J Urol 1992;147: 419–20.
86. Yokoyama O, Nagano K, Hirata A, et al. Clinical evaluation for voiding dysfunction in patients with cerebral palsy. Nippon Hinyokika Gakkai Zasshi 1989;80(4): 591–5.
87. Brodak PP, Scherz HC, Packer MG, et al. Is urinary tract screening necessary for patients with cerebral palsy? J Urol 1994;152:1586–7.

Establishing Access to Technology: An Evaluation and Intervention Model to Increase the Participation of Children with Cerebral Palsy

Elizabeth McCarty, OTR/L, ATP[a],*, Claire Morress, MEd, OTR/L, ATP[a,b]

KEYWORDS

- Cerebral palsy • Children • Participation • Assistive device
- Assistive technology • Model

The International Classification of Functioning, Disability and Health, known as the ICF,[1] provides a common language and classification system that focuses on health and health-related states instead of the consequences of disease, and represents a global paradigm shift in the way professionals view health and disability.[2,3] The ICF asserts that an individual's health and functioning should be measured by his or her participation in life situations, as opposed to the absence of disease. Participation is defined as "involvement in a life situation"[1] and it is an outcome of the interaction between the person with a health condition and the context in which he or she lives.[3] This has important implications for those working with individuals with conditions such as cerebral palsy (CP). CP is a chronic health condition that often results in participation restrictions in all areas of community and family life, including school, work, recreation, play, self-help, and mobility.[4–8] The ICF framework allows health professionals to expand their focus beyond impairment-based interventions and place equal value on those interventions that promote function and participation in life situations.[2] Thus,

[a] Aaron W. Perlman Center, Cincinnati Children's Hospital Medical Center, 3333 Burnet Avenue, Cincinnati, OH 45229, USA
[b] Department of Occupational Therapy, College of Social Sciences, Health and Education, Xavier University, 3800 Victory Parkway, Cincinnati, OH 45207, USA
* Corresponding author.
E-mail address: elizabeth.mccarty@cchmc.org (E. McCarty).

Phys Med Rehabil Clin N Am 20 (2009) 523–534
doi:10.1016/j.pmr.2009.05.001
1047-9651/09/$ – see front matter © 2009 Elsevier Inc. All rights reserved.

care delivery models should use a holistic approach that addresses the medical needs and the effects of the disability on function.

Therapeutic intervention for children with CP should include a systematic assessment of the physical abilities and the environmental/contextual constraints that impact participation, with an emphasis on how best to improve access to the environment and participation in all aspects of life. Assistive technology systems often present as the principal means for children with significant impairments and restrictions to effectively control their environment and engage in desired daily activities. Therapeutic challenges to implement successful assistive technology systems include establishing consistent access to or control of the assistive technology device and providing children with opportunities to use the device effectively in natural environments.

A multidisciplinary, family-centered approach to evaluate children's ability to access assistive technology and develop the skills necessary for successful use across all environments can be particularly effective. The aim of this article is to describe a 3-phase model of evaluation and intervention developed to maximize access to and control of assistive technology. The model relies on the continuous cycle of evaluation, intervention, and modification, which occurs in 1 or more of 3 sequential phases of skill acquisition: exploratory use, consistent use, and novel use. These phases incorporate developmental and ecologic considerations to provide interventions that are meaningful to the child and family across all environments. The literature confirms that assistive technology should be introduced early and evaluated frequently to maximize participation in activities that enhance early learning.[9] Early exposure to technology is indicated for some children with CP, and continual modifications of the technology and the intervention are needed as the child develops and acquires new skills through participation in his environment.

THEORETICAL FRAMEWORK

A combination of theoretical frameworks is suitable to guide interventions, with an emphasis on the developmental and ecologic factors that influence the functional skills of children with complex needs. Two specific theoretical approaches provide the framework for evaluating and establishing access in children with physical impairments, namely Piaget's theory of development and the Person-Environment-Occupation Model.[10]

Piaget viewed action and active engagement as instrumental processes in the cognitive and intellectual development of children.[11] Children with moderate to severe neurologic and developmental disabilities are often unable to explore or manipulate their natural environments independently.[12] Research has demonstrated that, by the age 4 years, a child with significant mobility restrictions may have already established a sense of learned helplessness and lack of motivation to explore the environment.[13,14] If children are not provided with developmentally appropriate opportunities for exploration and interaction, they are unable to actively construct and assimilate knowledge, thus development may be delayed.

It is a fundamental concept that children learn and develop by being active participants and not passive observers. Regardless of age, children benefit when a holistic view is taken and when focus is on increasing their active participation in all relevant environments (ie, parent-child interaction, preschool, school classroom, and community activities). When children with physical and neurologic impairments are given the opportunity to use an assistive technology device, they become more active participants and experience success and control over their environment. The 3-phase model for determining access recognizes that active, self-directed exploration is a key factor for development of skills in children. Therapists identify and use activities that are child-centered, developmentally appropriate, and motivating, and that provide opportunity for mastery and skill development.

A complementary ecological approach, such as the Person-Environment-Occupation Model,[10] focuses on person-environment interactions and provides therapists with a means of viewing and analyzing the occupational performance of children situated within their family and across all the environments where participation is desired. Intervention focuses on changing the child, the environment, or the task to maximize person-environment-occupation fit and occupational performance. Thus, this model provides an ideal framework for identifying the occupational performance issues of a child with cerebral palsy and targeting the area (person, environment, or task) that provides maximal effect and impact upon performance.

The concepts of the Person-Environment-Occupation Model[10] are readily incorporated into a therapeutic approach for evaluation of a child for access to technology (**Box 1**). The therapist should systematically evaluate the child's physical and cognitive skills, environmental barriers and facilitators (including family concerns), and the demands of the task (task analysis) to determine best fit for optimal device use. The emphasis is not solely on establishing normal movement patterns but on using the functional skills the child has and maximizing those skills through modifications

---

Box 1
General concepts for successful intervention

1. Allow the child time to experiment, explore, and have success. Children with disabilities often have processing deficits and decreased motor planning, and they require a longer time to respond to a task. If a child experiences success repeatedly, it is more likely that he/she will be motivated to continue. Before making the task more complicated, vary the activity at the same level of difficulty to allow for a greater chance of mastery.

2. If the child is required to perform a physically demanding task, the cognitive demands should be minimal. If the child is struggling to understand the concept of the task, it is more difficult to produce the physical response because both require significant energy.

3. The activity should be motivating and personalized to the likes of the child, if they are known. The more engaging the activity, the greater the reward for the child. Because it often takes significant efforts to produce a response, especially in the early phase of learning, the reward must be immediate and worth the effort.

4. The activity must be developmentally appropriate for the child. The developmental age (determined in the initial assessment) may be lower than the chronologic age. Cognitive match is important in that the activity will not be motivating if cognitively too difficult or too easy.

5. Once the control site and control interface have been established, integration into the child's environment is important. Allowing for the frequent use and opportunity in the child's environment is important for skill development and mastery. Providing a home set up gives the child the opportunity to gain skills in a familiar environment. Involving the family, so that they understand the value of the equipment and the functional benefits for their child to participate in their environment, helps to assure success.

6. Having a back-up access system is important to always allow the child the ability to participate. If a child is using a head mouse on their communication device, it is important to have a manual eye gaze board so that they can give quick responses. When the child is having significant medical issues or "bad body days" and is unable to access their typical system, having a low-tech system as a back-up will still allow the child to participate.

of task and environment to achieve optimal ability to use assistive technology and to participate in age-appropriate, meaningful, and motivating activities.

DEFINING ACCESS

The term "access" has been widely used in the assistive technology industry. Assistive technology is defined by Public Law 100-407 as "any item, piece of equipment, or product system, whether acquired commercially off the shelf, modified, or customized, that is used to increase or improve functional capabilities of individuals with disabilities."[15] Access refers to how the child is able to physically interact with and control his or her environment despite physical or cognitive deficits. This is often accomplished with assistive technology, thus the term access often refers to the method the child uses to control the assistive technology. There are 2 important terms to understand when evaluating for access: the control site and the control interface. The control site is the anatomic location or body part the child uses to physically activate the interface (switch, joystick, or adapted mouse), whereas the control interface is the hardware that controls the device.[15] The control site can be any anatomic location, for example, a hand, head, or index finger. The control interface may be a joystick, computer touch screen, custom keyboard, head mouse, or switch, to name a few. The general term "access" refers to the control site and the control interface, which, in combination, allow the child to interact with the assistive technology device and participate in the environment. For example, the child is physically able to extend their arm and hand (control site) to hit a button (interface) to open an automatic door (assistive technology device). Another example would be a child using her head (control site) to hit a switch (interface) to activate a computer program that reads a page of a book (assistive technology device).

When evaluating for access, a hierarchy of anatomic sites is recommended.[15] Hands and fingers are always the preferred anatomic site because of natural preference and their ability to manipulate objects with fine resolution and precision. The head and mouth are typically considered next because of the ability to use control interfaces that provide greater precision and control over devices, such as the head mouse, light beams, eye gaze, and mouth joysticks. The foot is a potential site when the child is unable to accurately use his or her hands, and it is likely that the feet can achieve fine resolution and range to control devices, such as a keyboard, mouse, or joystick, thereby providing accurate control of the devices. Generally the least physically affected body part or movement pattern, that is, the part of the body with movement over which the child has the greatest control, is preferred for access. The optimal control site or location is identified by thorough evaluation of the child's gross and fine motor control and functioning and is part of a more comprehensive multidisciplinary evaluation.

EVALUATION: THE FIRST STEP IN A CONTINUOUS CYCLE OF EVALUATION, INTERVENTION, AND MODIFICATION

A comprehensive initial evaluation is required to establish the needs of the child and family, the functional activities in which the child wishes to participate, and the skills and abilities the child has for accessing and using the desired assistive device(s). This is the first step in a continuous, dynamic cycle of assessment, intervention, and modification that may continue from preschool age until the child reaches adulthood (**Fig. 1**). During the evaluation, the team establishes the goal of the assistive technology (such as communication, mobility, or participation in educational activities or work),and the initial access site and control interface that will be used. Discipline-specific

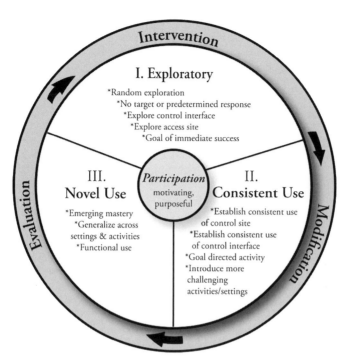

Fig. 1. Three-phase evaluation and intervention model: Depicts the phases of intervention and the continuous cycle of evaluation, intervention, and modification used to move the child toward functional device use and participation in daily activities.

evaluations focus on the developmental level, physical skills, language and cognitive abilities, postural control, motor planning, as well as sensory, auditory, and visual systems. The multidisciplinary treatment team may include an occupational therapist, speech pathologist, physical therapist, and developmental specialist. Specific information gleaned from this comprehensive assessment helps clinicians establish the child's baseline functional abilities and, for the purpose of access, helps to identify the most appropriate control site and control interface that will assist the child with participation. Additionally, it determines the developmental level of the child, so that the team can select the most motivating activities for initial intervention.

Because of the explosion of assistive technology devices available for purchase and the complex needs of individuals with cerebral palsy, it has become increasingly important to use a systematic feature match approach to evaluation. This means matching the needs and abilities of the consumer and the environments in which they live with the features of the device.[16] An important step in the process is to determine the child's and the family's needs, goals, expectations, and preferences and the environments in which they participate. This may be done through questionnaires mailed to the family, other professionals, and the school, and/or by face-to-face interview with the child and family. Consideration of personal factors is essential for continued device use and consumer satisfaction with equipment.[17] The family and child are instrumental in determining the functional needs and desired outcomes of the technology at every phase of evaluation and intervention. This is particularly important as the needs of the child, the family, and the environments in which they participate change with time as a result of growth and development.

The next step in establishing access to assistive technology is to determine a potential anatomic site and a specific control interface that the child will use to control the technology. This is done by incorporating the results of the comprehensive, multidisciplinary evaluation of client factors and performance skills with the family-needs assessment. The team must not lose sight of the environments in which the child and family participate, the supports and resources available to the family, or the preferences and goals of the child and family.

After identification of a potential access site and control interface, device trials are useful to confirm the outcome. It is important that at least 1 team member possess advanced and expert knowledge regarding assistive technology devices and applications, so that the team can select the most appropriate control interface and assistive technology device from the large number of options available. The physical requirements to operate the equipment vary depending upon the type of assistive technology being explored. Extended trials with the proposed equipment are a vital part of the evaluation because they can eliminate guesswork and reduce costly mistakes.

After the initial evaluation, the process of establishing reliable device use begins. Consistent with the Person-Environment-Occupation Model,[10] evaluation and intervention are viewed as ongoing, dynamic processes across time, and the child's ability to expand the use of the technology progresses along a developmental continuum, which is influenced by ever changing personal, environmental, and task-related factors. A 3-phase evaluation and intervention model for access to assistive technology, proceeding from exploratory use to consistent use and finally to novel use, can be aligned and modified with the child's developing skills and/or changing interests (see **Fig. 1**). Within each of the 3 phases, the team engages in a continuous cycle of evaluation and intervention and modifies treatment to allow for changes in the child or environment. It allows for progression and also for stepping back if needed. The emphasis is always on allowing the child's behavior and responses to guide and pace the intervention. Each phase represents a point along a developmental continuum of device use toward mastery.

THREE-PHASE EVALUATION AND INTERVENTION MODEL FOR DETERMINING ACCESS
Phase I. Exploratory Use

In the exploratory use phase, movements are purely experiential and are characterized by the children's drive to physically explore their world to discover relationships between their bodies and the environment. During this phase, the child is introduced to a control interface using the most appropriate control site (originally established through the initial evaluation). Through exploration, it may be determined that other control sites or interfaces may need to be considered. This phase is considered exploratory not only to explore the numerous options available for the control site and control interface but also to allow the child time to explore and act on his environment to discover outcomes of his/her actions. There is no required or predetermined response (**Fig. 2**).

During the phase of exploratory use, activities do not require a specific target or outcome. It is intended to be an opportunity to explore randomly without direction. This can be compared with a typical child given wooden blocks to manipulate without any knowledge or instruction that they can be used to build a tower. Instead, the child explores the shape, texture, or weight of the wooden blocks. He or she may throw the block or attempt to place 2 together. The initial movement (or device activation) may be purely random or imitative. This is part of the learning process. Once the child's actions cause something to happen that is of interest, it is more likely that he or she

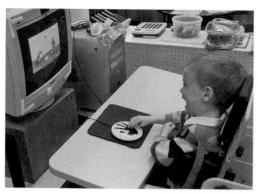

Fig. 2. Switch picture.

will try the movement pattern again. This repetition can lead to the development of more intentional, goal-directed device use.

For example, a child with physical disabilities may use a joystick or head mouse to activate a computer. During the phase of exploratory use, the therapist should provide computer games that do not require a left or right click; instead, the act of moving the joystick or head mouse in any direction should provide a visual and auditory response that is engaging and fun on the monitor. During this exploration, the child uses trial and error to learn how to manipulate the joystick or mouse and, at the same time, has the opportunity to explore space and movement. An immediate, motivating response to use the access method is crucial.

A child who is more physically challenged may require more time or additional control sites or control interfaces to establish the most appropriate equipment set up. Each time a new location is tried, the same exploratory environment should be provided. The child needs time to experiment, practice the motor control, and experience success. It is important for the therapist to resist the urge to move too quickly through this phase.

The selection of activities is important to the successful use of assistive technology in the phase of exploratory use. Using activities that provide auditory and visual feedback (such as switch toys) can be motivating for a child; however, they may not hold the child's interest. Consideration of the child's cognitive and developmental level, determined during the initial evaluation, is important in selection of activities that are motivating in this and subsequent phases. The therapist should be creative and may have to set up playful environments that allow for exploration of objects and space. This can be challenging when the child is only able to use a single switch for access. Examples might include having animal races with switch toys or having the toy dog fetch the ball and go into the doghouse. Computer software is also an excellent resource to allow for varied activities that offer visual and auditory feedback. Using a power wheelchair programmed to spin in 1 direction allows the child to experience movement while still learning the same motor pattern required for hitting a single switch. Peer interaction is a powerful motivator, and it provides the opportunity for social interaction and communication.

Key to successful technology use in the exploratory phase is to allow the child time to explore the new technology and to provide motivating and varied activities that do not require a specific outcome. Moving the child too quickly through this phase may cause frustration because children need time to practice these new skills. Giving too much verbal prompting at this level should be resisted because the child will learn best through doing, with natural consequences.

Phase II. Consistent Use

The phase of consistent use is characterized by goal-directed use of the control interface and exploratory use of the device for different ends. Children require multiple opportunities to practice newly learned skills across natural environments to establish consistent, goal-directed use of the control interface for engagement in functional skills. During this phase, more challenging activities can be introduced, and the activity can be more self-directed. The child continues to require immediate, motivating feedback and success (**Fig. 3**).

For example, a child using a joystick may be required to click on an object and move it to another part of the screen. A head mouse or switch user may have 2 choices at first, and each choice offers immediate feedback. As the child masters 2 choices, a third and forth can be added. The demands of the task should be slowly and selectively increased to challenge the child and build skills for success. Use of creative, motivating activities continues to be key to maintaining the child's interest.

A viable control site and control interface should have been identified and established during the exploratory phase. During this phase, this site is used consistently and repeatedly across different environments and for different activities to establish reliable, accurate, and efficient access to the technology. Additionally, the child should be introduced to more functional use of the device in natural environments. The child is now encouraged to take the device home to practice; however, activities should be carefully selected to fit into families' routines and natural occupations, and family members must be adequately trained in the use and set-up of the device before taking it home. Use is strictly limited to predetermined times and activities so as not to over-challenge the child or family.

During this phase the child learns to master the control site and control interface, while starting to be challenged with higher demands of the activities. The therapist carefully grades and adapts the task and the environment to foster skill development and greater independence, while continuing to meet the needs of the child and the family. These activities still require immediate feedback, and the child must experience success.

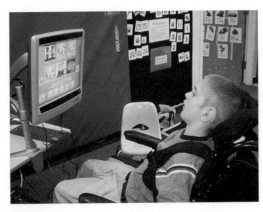

Fig. 3. Exploring eye gaze.

Phase III. Novel Use

In the phase of novel use, the child has gained mastery of the control site and control interface and learns to conceptualize and generalize device use across multiple settings for a variety of different purposes. The child learns to use the device for novel ends and requires fewer modifications to the set up and the environment. The child is able to initiate a response, answer a question, or activate a toy with less assistance and fewer cues. They are able to participate in a functional activity of their choice and provide novel responses (**Fig. 4**).

Activities can be introduced that require additional concentration or duration of time to complete. The device can also be used in multiple environments. For example, an augmentative communication device user can participate in the pledge of allegiance at school by having the pledge divided into multiple cell locations on the device. The same child might go to a restaurant and use his or her communication device to select a meal. A child playing a familiar computer game should be able to use the same strategies for unfamiliar games. Instead of being limited to a controlled environment, the child in this phase begins to use their control interface to operate more than 1 type of device. For example, the child who accesses a communication device using a head mouse can also use it to play a computer game.

GENERAL CONSIDERATIONS WHEN USING THE 3-PHASE MODEL

Not all children demonstrate the capacity to achieve all stages of device use, and each child progresses through the stages at a different rate. Some children may always require a structured environment and may never be able to use the technology in multiple environments. In some cases, the activities may be used for leisure only and provide the opportunity for independent play, whereas for others a device may be used to write a school paper.

Procuring equipment can be done during any phase of the intervention and can change as the child progresses. An example of this process would be that for a child whose initial evaluation determined that a single switch placed at the left temple was the optimal access method. During the exploratory phase, the child used simple cause and effect games that produced sounds and visual images via the computer. After a week of intervention, the child demonstrated difficulty using the switch, yet the

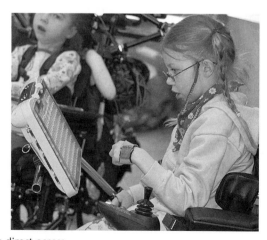

Fig. 4. Emily using direct access.

placement was still considered the most optimal. Following the evaluation-intervention-modification approach, the team ultimately recommended a larger switch with increased sensitivity. The child was then given the opportunity to explore this control interface using the same computer games. The team did not advance the child to the second phase (consistent use) until the child was able to use the switch with ease. This child might never move beyond the ability to hit a switch for cause and effect or may take a long period of time to advance.

The 3-phase model allows therapists to monitor the continuous changes in the child that occur as a result of therapeutic intervention and to accommodate these changes as they occur. Continual evaluation also permits the therapist to incorporate any environmental changes or medical interventions that may occur that affect the child's ability to participate.

INDEPENDENT PLAY OPPORTUNITIES

Providing opportunities for independent play is important for a child's learning and development when advancing through the 3 phases. Children with disabilities can fall into a cycle of learned helplessness. They can become passive and unmotivated[13] because of lack of opportunity to participate in their environment. This can result in lack of interest and failure to develop the skills they need to interact with their environment.[9] Providing independent play activities with the most appropriate access method gives the child an opportunity to explore a newly learned skill to gain proficiency. In addition, it gives the child a chance to explore without the verbal or physical commands of another person. Although this may be difficult for family members to allow because of their own needs to provide care for the child, with time this is an excellent opportunity for both the child and the parent. Independent play is incorporated into each phase of the 3-phase model. As the child gains success within each level and mastery with the technology, independence is likely to continue to increase.

FUTURE DIRECTIONS

Although research confirms that children with CP experience limitations in participation in all areas, including school, recreation, and leisure activities,[4–8] and assistive technology is widely used with children with CP, there is little research to support specific clinical intervention strategies to maximize participation and assistive technology use in this population. This is partly due to the complexity of the construct of participation and difficulty in obtaining homogeneous groups for comparison. Most intervention is therefore based on expert knowledge and clinical experience. The 3-phase model of progression through exploratory, consistent, and novel use phases of assistive technology by children with CP is guided by sound theoretical principles and best practice and has yielded desired clinical outcomes. However, there is a need for systematic research to investigate the efficacy of this approach and to better document the outcomes relating to functional performance, as well as client satisfaction and impact on health-related quality of life.

SUMMARY

Children with a diagnosis of CP may have significant physical limitations that prevent exploration and full participation in the environment. Limited experiences can lead to secondary impairments and complications, such as delayed development and learned helplessness. Assistive technology systems can provide opportunities for children with physical limitations to interact with their world, enabling play, communication, and daily living skills. Efficient access to and control of the technology is critical for successful use; however, establishing consistent access is often difficult because of the nature of the movement patterns exhibited by children with CP. The 3-phase model of evaluation and intervention to establish access to assistive technology for children with physical disabilities allows progression from exploratory use through consistent use and, finally, novel use. This model uses all options for success, including promoting the use of assistive technology to develop compensatory skills, modifying the demands of the environment, and supporting changes in the child's performance and physical abilities. Determining a child's best means of access for maximum participation, establishing consistent use of the equipment, and using an intervention approach that provides opportunity for constant reevaluation and modification is critical for implementing successful assistive technology systems for children with CP.

REFERENCES

1. World Health Organization. International classification of functioning, disability and health (ICF). Geneva: World Health Organization; 2001.
2. Rosenbaum P, Stewart D. The World Health Organization classification of functioning, disability, and health: a model to guide clinical thinking, practice and research in the field of cerebral palsy. Semin Pediatr Neurol 2004;11(1):5–10.
3. World Health Organization. Towards a common language for functioning, disability, and health: ICF. Available at: http://www.who.int/classifications/icf/training/icfbeginnersguide.pdf. 2002. Accessed June 12, 2007.
4. Beckung E, Hagberg G. Neuroimpairments, activity limitations, and participation restrictions in children with cerebral palsy. Dev Med Child Neurol 2002;44: 309–16.
5. Brown M, Gordon W. Impact of impairment on activity patterns of children. Arch Phys Med Rehabil 1987;68:828–32.
6. Kerr C, McDowell B, McDonough S. The relationship between gross motor function and participation restriction in children with cerebral palsy: an exploratory analysis. Child Care Health Dev 2006;33(1):22–7.
7. Law M, King G, King S, et al. Patterns of participation in recreational and leisure activities among children with complex physical disabilities. Dev Med Child Neurol 2006;48:337–42.
8. Pollock N, Stewart D. A survey of activity patterns and vocational readiness of young adults with physical disabilities. Can J Rehabil 1990;4(1):17–26.
9. Swinth Y. Assistive technology: low technology, computers, electronic aids for daily living, and augmentative communication. In: Case-Smith J, editor. Occupational therapy for children. 5th edition. St Louis (MO): Elsevier; 2005. p. 615–56.
10. Law M, Cooper B, Strong S, et al. The person-environment-occupation model: a transactive approach to occupational performance. Can J Occup Ther 1996; 63:9–23.
11. Bybee RW, Sund RB. Piaget for educators. 2nd edition. Columbus (OH): Charles E Merrill; 1982.
12. Deitz J, Swinth Y, White O. Powered mobility and preschoolers with complex developmental delays. Am J Occup Ther 2002;56:86–96.
13. Butler C. Wheelchair toddlers. In: Furamasu J, editor. Pediatric powered mobility: developmental perspectives, technical issues, clinical approaches. Arlington (VA): RESNA Press; 1997. p. 1–6.

14. Wright-Ott C. The transitional powered mobility aid, a new concept and tool for early mobility. In: Furamasu J, editor. Pediatric powered mobility: developmental perspectives, technical issues, clinical approaches. Arlington (VA): RESNA Press; 1997. p. 58–69.
15. Cook A, Hussey S. Assistive technologies: principles and practice. 2nd edition. St Louis (MO): Mosby; 2002.
16. Sherer MJ. Matching consumers with appropriate assistive technologies. In: Olson D, DeRuyter F, editors. Clinicians' guide to assistive technology. St Louis (MO): Mosby; 2002. p. 3–13.
17. Scherer M, Jutai J, Fuhrer M, et al. A framework for modeling the selection of assistive technology devices (ATDs). Disability and rehabilitation. Assist Technol 2007;2(1):1–8.

Access to Employment and Economic Independence in Cerebral Palsy

Susie Rutkowski, MEd[a], Erin Riehle[a,b],*

KEYWORDS

- Project search • Disability • Employment • Partnerships
- Transition • Cerebral palsy • Cognitive challenges

"It's Monday … everyone works on Monday." So says the familiar line of one of our favorite movies "Dave." Do you look forward to work on Monday? Do you look forward to the job itself, the people, and the pay? Do you think about your job over the weekend with dread, frustration, or excitement?

For many of us, work defines us, or at least a big part of us. At a party or picnic people ask, "What do you do?" meaning "Where do you work?" and "Do you like it?" The other underlying message is "How do you contribute?"

But what if you don't work? Not because you are retired, or a student, or staying home raising children, but because you have never had the opportunity to work. The employment statistics for people with disabilities are dismal and particularly low for those with cerebral palsy (CP). Michelsen and colleagues reported that only 29% of 819 participants with CP aged 21 to 35 years identified from Denmark's unique Danish Cerebral Palsy Registry were competitively employed, in comparison with 82% of controls, and 5% of those who were studying.[1] Participants with CP generally had a lower annual income than controls. Participants with hemiplegia had the highest employment rate (46%), followed by those with diplegia (26%), and among those with quadriplegia, only 12% were competitively employed. Among the participants with CP who were able to walk, the severity of motor impairment was found to be only a minor influence. The odds ratio for not being competitively employed was 22.5 for those individuals with a developmental quotient (DQ) of 50 to 85 in comparison with those with a DQ over 85. Completing education had training and employment

[a] Project SEARCH, Cincinnati Children's Hospital Medical Center, ML 5030, 3333 Burnet Avenue, Cincinnati, OH 45229, USA
[b] Disability Services, Cincinnati Children's Hospital Medical Center, ML 5030, 3333 Burnet Avenue, Cincinnati, OH 45229, USA
* Corresponding author. Disability Services, Cincinnati Children's Hospital Medical Center, ML 5030, 3333 Burnet Avenue, Cincinnati, OH 45229.
E-mail address: erin.riehle@cchmc.org (E. Riehle).

Phys Med Rehabil Clin N Am 20 (2009) 535–547
doi:10.1016/j.pmr.2009.06.003
1047-9651/09/$ – see front matter © 2009 Elsevier Inc. All rights reserved.
pmr.theclinics.com

implications. Fifty-one percent of participants obtained secondary school education, whereas 45% of participants with CP, compared with 5% of controls, never passed an examination in lower secondary school. Type and severity of CP differed substantially with educational attainment, but even among individuals with hemiplegia, only 50% had education beyond lower secondary school compared with 77% of controls. Participants with education beyond lower secondary school often had mild CP. Rather simple clinical characteristics in early childhood seem to predict future employment. Motor disability, which is the defining characteristic of CP and the focus of much of the rehabilitation effort, seems to be of relatively minor influence across all types of CP. In the Danish study, significant predictors of not being competitively employed were severity of cognitive impairment, type of cerebral palsy, presence of epilepsy, and severe motor impairment.

A literature review of employment outcomes in CP yields limited studies. Most available data are from studies with small numbers and varied work outcomes that show an overall low employment statistics. In the United States the National Health Interview Survey, conducted by the Census Bureau/National Center for Health Statistics, is a very large longitudinal study, however its statistics are reported in relation to the general population of people with disabilities and not broken down by persons with specific impairments such as CP. A small study of male workers with CP (8) focused on those using augmentative and alternative communication (AAC) with college level education.[2] Although interesting predictors were identified, the lack of data available on young adults with significant cognitive challenges is still highlighted.

An estimated 764,000 children and adults in the United States exhibit one or more symptoms of cerebral palsy. The range of motor function impairment varies widely from mild isolated impairment of motor abilities to severe disabilities in motor, speech, cognition and epilepsy. As persons with cerebral palsy age, they may develop secondary conditions (see also the article by Murphy and colleagues in this issue). Daily living skills may become more difficult over time. Secondary conditions and decreasing overall function may significantly affect the amount of technical and personal support a person with cerebral palsy needs to be successful in an integrated working environment for the a prolonged period of time. The three areas of functioning that are critical to job seeking and work performance are self-care, physical functioning/mobility and communication. Job seeking is severely affected because of intense personal needs and perceptions of employers and human resources personnel. A person with intense personal care needs may use some of his earnings to pay for someone to help him get ready for work, assist him during the job, meet after-work needs and even assist with navigating the complicated maze of government work incentives. Low tech and high tech solutions can often make it possible for someone to be productively employed and overcome deficits in these three areas.

The national advocacy organization United Cerebral Palsy (UCP), in their Annual Case for Inclusion 2008, developed a vision for persons with CP with intellectual and developmental disabilities containing 4 commitments:

○ People with disabilities will live in and participate in their communities
○ People with disabilities will have satisfying lives and valued social roles
○ People with disabilities will have sufficient access to needed support and control over that support so that the assistance they receive contributes to lifestyles they desire
○ People will be safe and healthy in the environments in which they live

Even though these commitments have been articulated in a number of legislative, administrative, and judicial statements describing national policy, they do not specifically mention employment. One can speculate that the goal of competitive employment is implied in the first 3 commitments. It would seem critical for any prominent national policy organization for persons with CP to articulate explicit strategies for increasing employment opportunities and lead the way to impact employment outcomes positively.

In his review of the health and well-being of adults with CP, Liptak[3] observed that, in our culture, well-being has traditionally been defined to include completing formal education, entering the work force, living independently, having romantic relationships, participating in recreation and/or leisure, driving a car, and enjoying social group encounters. Literature and experience indicate that many young adults with CP are not achieving these common accomplishments.

This article reviews the relevant literature; conclusions are drawn and recommendations made to improve the employment outcomes for youth with CP in their transition to adult life. It is widely recognized that youth with disabilities have articulated that their top priority is employment. What are some of the reasons why they are not being successful in that endeavor?

BARRIERS TO EMPLOYMENT OF PERSONS WITH CEREBRAL PALSY

When most job seekers are making decisions on which job offer to accept, they consider factors such as quality of match for their life, their skill set, and their knowledge. For youth and adults with disabilities, these decisions are much more dynamic. They may need to consider additional factors such as the availability of specialized or public transportation, access to assistive technology (AT), effects on their disability benefits, and overall attitudes and perceptions of people toward those with disabilities. Attitudinal and cultural barriers continue to exacerbate environmental constraints such as inaccessibility and discrimination continues to define the disability experience.[4] For those with significant physical challenges such as CP, these considerations are more critical. Individuals with severe CP may not be able to perform simple work tasks without accommodations or even a personal care assistant. Additional challenges include access to appropriate training and skill acquisition leading to adequate preparation for work. Acquisition of appropriate behavior and social skills are additional factors. Young people with CP may be less socially active (and sometimes less socially appropriate) than their typical peers. As they get older, they may lack the social competence to seek and maintain personal friendships and to seek needed services. Coupled with the other factors, this creates barriers to successful employment. Individuals without disability, in contrast, become more socially active after school age. Wadsworth and Harper noted that for adults with and without disability, the lack of ability to function socially is a very important factor associated with failure to obtain employment and difficulty in adapting.[5]

Expectation level is another key factor in employment outcomes of youth with CP. Are parents, teachers, family members, and the young people themselves expecting a competitive job when they graduate from high school? How often does a family member say to a young child with a disability, "What are you going to be when you grow up?" Does the high school guidance counselor ask a teen with CP, "What are you going to do when you graduate? How will you prepare for the job that you want?" Instead, educators are often forced to concentrate on high stakes testing, required classes for graduation, physical accommodations, and development of educational goals that do not prepare the young person for a successful transition to adult life and competitive employment. Work-study programs too often concentrate on traditional jobs in food service, which are often not suitable for youth with CP.

High expectations from families, schools, and society that young adults with disabilities will enter the competitive workforce would drive government policy, create appropriate training programs, and result in more outcomes of young adults with CP moving seamlessly from high school to a job that matches their interests, preparation, and skill level.

Stevenson and colleagues[6] found that teachers, care assistants, or others involved with the daily activities of young people with CP rated the prospects for employment for most of them as poor or rather poor. These young people still in school ranked the importance of getting a job a top priority. The mothers of 27 young people (36.5%) considered their children unfit for employment. Just over half of the others indicated that help was needed in forming a realistic plan for the future of their child, but most of them did not know who would help in forming such a plan.

In a study by Murphy and colleagues,[8] involving 125 adults with CP in 2000, 21% were involved in competitive employment. Based on their outcomes, the investigators provided advice for adolescents with CP entering high school:

- Set your own goals
- Do not accept unnecessary school restrictions because of your disability
- Seek out successful adult role models with a similar disability
- Recognize that feelings of identity crisis are common in all adolescents

Another barrier to setting high expectations for employment of youth with CP is that society often regards disability due to CP as a medical issue. When this occurs, the focus may become the cure or treatment of the symptoms of the disability instead of the preparation and training of the young person to develop competitive and marketable skills. When the individual with CP is a "patient," it is difficult to change the paradigm to the individual as a "worker." Cultural perceptions and systemic changes need to take place before employment outcomes for youth with CP improve.

Another study warranting attention is that of McNaughton and colleagues of a small population of 8 males with CP, aged between 30 and 57 years, with education ranging from completion of some college credits to completion of a doctoral degree, who used AAC and were employed full time.[2] Through participation in a focus group conducted on the Internet, this small group provided a rich array of recommendations that have application across the age spectrum to youth with disabilities. Some of the benefits of employment included accomplishing personal goals, increasing self-esteem, putting their minds and education to use, making a positive contribution, and achieving financial benefits and positive experiences at work. Also of significance were the negative impacts of employment: physical demands, time demands, and societal prejudice. Their list of personal characteristics, as well as accommodations and supports for successful employment, are applicable to youth with CP and cognitive issues. Factors identified as key to preparation for successful employment included appropriate education, career exploration, and vocational experiences. Community networks, government policies, and computer technology were identified as important supports for obtaining employment. Personal characteristics such as a strong commitment to employment, work ethic, determination, persistence, and time management skills were key factors. Technology, supportive coworkers, personal care assistance, and family support were described as important supports for maintaining employment. These study subjects provided some very insightful recommendations to educators:

- Be aware of the students' abilities and assist them to reach their full potential
- Prepare them with productive skills

- Expand students' knowledge of job options
- Have high expectations
- Design adequate training in job search skills

EMPLOYMENT STATISTICS FOR EDUCATION AND EMPLOYMENT OF PEOPLE WITH DISABILITIES

Almost all of the research shows that the employment rate for persons with disabilities is low. A variety of different reports using diverse measures all have similar outcomes. From *The State of Disability in America:*[4] According to the US Census Bureau's Current Population Survey, the 2005 employment rate for working-aged Americans with a work disability was 22%, whereas the employment rate for working-aged Americans without a disability was 76%. The Census Bureau's American Community Survey found that 38% of working-aged Americans with disabilities and 78% of working-aged Americans without disabilities were employed in 2005. The Census Bureau's Survey of Income and Program Participation found that 45% of working-aged Americans with severe disabilities were employed in 2002, compared with 88% of working-aged Americans without disabilities. Men with disabilities worked one-third as many weeks during 2002 as men without disabilities. Women with disabilities worked about one-fourth as many weeks as women without disabilities. The data offer only a recent snapshot at the end of a long slow decline in the employment rate of adults with disabilities. Government statistics and academic studies consistently show that employment rates for men and women with disabilities have declined steadily since the recession of 1991 to 1992.

Studies on employment of people with disabilities, although not specific to those with CP, are inclusive of them, and directly correlate with the data associated with income and poverty.[2] In 2005, the median annual household income of working-aged Americans without disabilities was $61,500. The median annual household income of working-aged Americans with disabilities was $35,000, a deficit of more than $26,000. Adult workers with disabilities were almost 3 times as likely to live in poverty as people without disabilities. Individuals with disabilities are more likely to live in poverty and to be dependent on government support. They are less likely to have positive educational opportunities and outcomes, to be employed, or to own a home. In 2005, more than 37 million Americans lived in poverty, about 40% of whom had a disability. Poor families are twice as likely to have a child with a disability and 50% more likely to have a child with a severe disability. Adults with disabilities were more than twice as likely to have less education than a high school degree than were adults without disabilities. Twenty-two percent of students with disabilities failed to graduate high school compared with 9% of students without disabilities.

EMPLOYMENT STATISTICS FOR EDUCATION AND EMPLOYMENT OF PEOPLE WITH CP

Approximately 90% of children with CP in the United States survive into their 20s and beyond (compared with 98% of the general population of children), thus issues related to adult participation are relevant and should be anticipated. Several studies have found diminished participation in society among adults who have CP. In their study in Denmark, Michelsen and colleagues[7] found that 55% of 416 adult participants with CP aged 29 to 35 years had no competitive employment, partner, or children compared with 4% of a comparison group. In this study, no sign of increased social integration was reported over 2 to 3 decades. In an earlier report by this same group of investigators,[1] among 819 adults with CP aged 21 to 35 years, the percentage of competitively employed adults varied by type of CP: hemiplegia 46%, diplegia 26%, and quadriplegia 12%, with 29% total employment for participants with CP compared with 82% for the control group. The employment rate has consistently been reported to be lower in adults who have CP than in comparable adults without disabilities. In a study from Minnesota, Murphy and colleagues[8] found 53% of adults with CP to be competitively employed; however, 22% of these individuals earned an income high enough that advancement would cause financial loss through termination of disability benefits. These investigators noted that this rate is higher than that previously reported for achievement of competitive employment and independent living for adults with CP with moderate to severe disability. Between 1983 and 1996 the employment rate for all adults with CP in the United States was reported to be 42%.[4] More advanced rehabilitation technology, better home support services, and legal mandates in education and environmental access have been proposed as facilitators of positive changes impacting employment outcomes for persons with CP in the United States.[8] Employment rates for youth under the Individuals with Disabilities Education Act (IDEA) are twice those of older adults with similar disabilities and the percentage of college freshman reporting disabilities has more than tripled since 1978.[4]

MAJOR LEGISLATION AFFECTING EDUCATION AND EMPLOYMENT FOR PEOPLE WITH DISABILITIES

In 1868 the 14th Amendment was ratified by the states, codifying into law the foundation for equality: that no state shall "deny to any person within its jurisdiction the equal protection of the laws." Nevertheless, it would still take more than a century before American schools were opened to children with disabilities. As a result of advocacy efforts, mostly by parents, Congress acted in 1975 and passed the Education for All Handicapped Children Act, commonly known as Public Law 94-142. This law, which revolutionized the educational environment for children with disabilities, mandated that children with disabilities were guaranteed a "free and appropriate public education" in the "least restrictive environment," tailored to their individual unique needs. It protected the rights of children with disabilities and their families against discrimination in provision of educational services and assisted states and localities in implementing integrated educational environments with federal funding. The law has been reauthorized several times, most recently in December 2004 with new emphasis on transition outcomes.

The Americans with Disabilities Act (ADA) was passed on July 26, 1990. This landmark piece of legislation on disability rights mandates equal access to employment in many large employment venues. Some small, privately owned businesses are exempt. However, the spirit and letter of the ADA can be felt across all industry sectors and sizes.

President Clinton issued an Executive Order in July 2000 that requires federal executive branch agencies and departments to hire an additional 100,000 individuals with disabilities over the following 5 years. Even though this never occurred, public awareness of the problem of underemployment of people with disabilities was increased; there has been subsequent, more recent discussion to move further in the direction of implementation.

CURRENT CHALLENGES

In spite of some progress indicating some signs of optimism for the future, limited educational opportunities and outcomes, rampant poverty, high unemployment, and dependence on public benefits continue to prevent many people with disabilities from achieving independent and productive lives.[4] Evidence presented in the earlier sections supports this. The underlying reasons and solutions are multifactorial. Youth with disabilities have diverse challenges with limitations in options to meet their needs. Some communities do a great job creating services and supports to meet their challenges. Yet it often appears that 1 step is taken forward and 2 steps backward in implementing solutions.

There are several major challenges that must be addressed to create successful scenarios for youth with disabilities:

- Complicated government programs and policies such as Medicaid, Social Security and Vocational Rehabilitation
- Lack of educationally appropriate work experience programs
- Low expectations on the part of society, schools, and families
- Inadequate transition planning and/or not enough community resources

The Medicaid and Social Security benefits system is excessively complicated. Even though work incentives exist, most families cannot use them because they either do not know about them to inquire at the Social Security Office, the employees that families encounter are not trained adequately to assist them, or the process of use is cumbersome and time consuming for clients and families. Families are often afraid to try accessing the benefits system; if there are changes in work status, there is the possibility of receiving overpayments or of losing benefits altogether. If significant disability is associated with health care issues, having medical insurance is imperative. Relying on government insurance programs and keeping under the income limit so medical benefits are not lost, keeps people with disability in a cycle of poverty unless the family has additional sources of unearned income. This affects the potential of people with CP from achieving a common goal: living and working independently.

For youth with CP there are numerous challenges within the educational system in their transition to employment. Even though the new IDEA 2004 has focused attention on this transition and emphasizes the schools' responsibility in this area, there is no new funding to accompany the mandates. "No Child Left Behind" requires schools to undertake testing and reporting, which takes time away from implementing meaningful programs that could result in improved preparation for the youth and appropriate skill acquisition for employment and economic independence. Studies and experience show that the more involved families are in the special education process, the better their transition outcomes. However, most schools do not have the funding to hire parent mentors who might help at-risk families navigate the system. There are divergent research outcomes and practices related to inclusion of students with significant cognitive challenges into all regular classes versus allowing them to participate in a functional curriculum and on-the-job training, which facilitates career exploration and employment. There are few appropriate educational training options that prepare youth with significant cognitive and physical challenges for nontraditional employment. Work-based learning programs not only develop technical skills but also create critical thinking and problem solving skills, teamwork, and appropriate social skills. Workers who have both the specific work skills and other soft skills are more likely to be hired and have longevity and career advancement. Students with cognitive and physical disabilities, including many with CP, already "stick out;" they need every opportunity to become part of the fabric of a work environment and develop natural paths for success.

Aside from barriers related to educational and governmental programs, attitudes and expectations may be severe deterrents to achieving employment. Murphy and colleagues[8] found a high percentage (84%) of young adults with CP who felt that their parents overprotected them. As children, more freedom and risk taking should be allowed, comparable with that allowed for peers without disabilities, as appropriate. In 1975, Marc Gold, the founder of supported employment, stated: "Low expectancy on the part of society is the single most critical deterrent to programs for persons with severe disability." This is still too often true 34 years later, as reflected in the findings of recent studies cited earlier.

The federal special educational mandate states that transition planning should begin at least by age 16 years through the Individualized Education Program process. There is also a mandate that vocational rehabilitation services work in tandem with the educational system to provide employment training opportunities. With continued poor outcomes, we are not doing a good job in either transition planning, execution, or employment results. Although some communities have many options and coordinated efforts, many (especially in rural areas) do not have adequate planning, partnerships, or programs to promote transition and competitive employment. Programs such as Vocational Rehabilitation (VR) are not consistent from state to state or even within regions. Because VR counselors can be autonomous, youth may receive very different services. As a result of increasing numbers of youth seeking services and budget cuts, many states have gone to "Order of Selection" so that transition-aged youth can apply, but many are put on waiting lists and fail to receive timely support.

POTENTIAL SOLUTIONS: BEST PRACTICES AND PARTNERSHIPS

"People with disabilities have the right to choose a path toward education and employment. However, while freedom of choice is given, the right to work is earned. Earning the right to work is dependent upon the student's preparation.."[9]

Young people with disabilities have many entitlements, educational services, and programs available for a "free and appropriate public education." From the age of 3 to 21 years, schools and families should work together to prepare the youth for a successful transition to the adult world. It is imperative at some stage that the students take major responsibility in the planning and implementation of their own goals, classes, and programs. If we are going to have high expectations of young people with cognitive and physical disabilities joining the competitive work force, their role in the preparation is critical. A strong work ethic has been identified as one of the most effective factors in maintaining successful employment. A second essential factor vitally important in the workplace, when seeking and then maintaining employment, is efficient, effective, and appropriate communication for work and social purposes.[2]

In evaluating transition practices, it is useful to incorporate consideration of 3 common elements of transition models: preparation, linkage, and connection or reception. Preparing the student with moderate to severe disabilities for transition to adulthood requires education and experiences that include social skills and skills for independent living as well as academic and technical career training. Life skills are an important part of transition education for students with all levels of disabilities. These skills include training in the areas of social competence, employability, and participation in the community, and should be taught in a variety of settings including the classroom, the community, and the workplace.[10] We do not live or work in isolation. In any endeavor, it is necessary to involve other people and organizations to use resources and ideas. Our economy and culture demand it. In order to make a difference, we have to join forces and bring together all the needed supports and services to ensure that students are adequately prepared. Making linkages is critical: a variety of services are needed at the same time; it is not reasonable or cost efficient to duplicate services.

As noted by McNaughton and colleagues[2] community networks, particularly family and friends, play a critical role in opening the door to potential employment opportunities. Generally, parents are involved and are usually very supportive during the transition process. They can bring their own set of resources to help meet the goal of their child's employment. One linkage often ignored in the transition and educational processes is business. Large employers are often seen as the end result (employment) and less often as part of the process. As we have seen in the current global economic crisis, businesses (especially big businesses) affect the local community and the world. We also know that large businesses are the ones most affected by diversity initiatives and disability policy, for example, the ADA, whereas small organizations (those hiring less than 15 workers) are exempt from the employment provisions in Title I of the ADA. Large businesses (hospitals, banks, retail companies) are seen as leaders in the community. They are often eager to connect with schools and community partners to make a positive difference and discover a talented new pool of workers.

As 1 best practice example Project SEARCH in Cincinnati, Ohio, created a business-led partnership that also included partners from education, rehabilitation, and long-term support. It has been replicated in a variety of industry sectors and geographic locales. It combines preparation in employability skills with career exploration and real work experiences. Students have an active role in choosing three internships and gain constant feedback through their instructor, a community job coach, and a coworker in the business. This is not simulated work that might be established in a classroom or sheltered work environment. "Real time" work is being performed and provides the vehicle for acquiring critical core skills needed for a competitive work environment.

Among the issues previously discussed were perceptions, attitudes, and expectations. Partnering with a business-led program will begin to have an impact on the organization with a positive presence of disability and create the cultural change necessary for overcoming stereotypes about workers with disabilities. Programs such as Project SEARCH show that young people with disabilities, including CP, can demonstrate necessary skills, modify their performance, and articulate their successes and challenges so that the business sees young people with cognitive and physical disabilities as a talent stream that meets their labor needs. For the last 3 school years (2005–2006, 2006–2007, 2007–2008) Project SEARCH has averaged a 77% job placement outcome. There is also strong evidence of a paradigm shift in the business culture of the host organizations toward welcoming workers with significant cognitive and physical disabilities. Project SEARCH has succeeded in part because it partnered existing organizations in the community and braided existing funding. Beyond start-up costs, the program is sustainable. Business, education, and rehabilitation are working together (not duplicating services) to create a seamless system of training and supporting individuals with CP and other disabilities. Students doing real work through internships mutually benefit businesses and trainees. Hospitals host nursing and physical therapy students in internships and preceptorships from many types of educational institutions. City and state governments host college interns from business and public management programs. Banks host intern leadership programs to recruit the best financial students from local colleges. The organization of the Project SEARCH program makes sense to business and to young people with disabilities. It also takes the typical work-study model several steps further along the continuum. For many technical career schools, it provides a mechanism to serve students who might not be successful in a typical workforce development program. Rehabilitation and other long-term support agencies can partner and share the costs of job coaching and work accommodations. Employability skills are built into the program, through the curriculum and the internship sites. Students are immersed in the program all day, every day for an entire school year, creating a greater impact on their own learning and within the host business. In November 2006, Disability World reported that Project SEARCH is doing more than providing valuable work experiences for students.[11] It is managing and changing corporate culture and the receptivity of workplaces to employ people with disabilities.

Students with AT needs in the workplace will reap the benefits of others. Technology will be created for groups such as veterans and astronauts that will be eventually used by youth with AT needs. Revolutionary advances in AT are occurring every day.

Research and experience show that employment programs for individuals with disabilities have better outcomes for people at a younger age than with older adults. Among the factors are the human and financial benefits from schools and families. Once a student graduates, the support systems that provide educators, therapists, curriculum, programs, AT, and other resources that surround the student are no longer available. Because of the emphasis on positive transition outcomes in IDEA 2004, many school districts have hired transition specialists. Many communities have organized transition teams with the school district, taking the lead. Other agencies such as VR often partner schools to share the responsibility of transition and rehabilitation. VR has connections to Supplemental Security Income or Social Security Disability Income benefit information and can help navigate that system to maximize earned income. Families with their networks and connections are often very involved in the transition years, but that support often decreases after school completion.

Youth with disabilities become less social and have more difficulty making necessary connections as they get older. Creation of successful programs for transition-aged youth takes advantage of their energy and positive excitement about training (as well as mandatory attendance requirements) to become a successful contributing member of the community. If students with disabilities graduate and do not enter the workforce or participate in sheltered employment, they generally have difficulty gaining competitive skills and finding typical employment.

Based on the literature and on recommendations and information from people with CP and other disabilities, from national organizations and from researchers, 1 repeated theme was that youth with disabilities need to be more involved in their own education, training, and goal setting. There are four guiding principles of self-determination or self-advocacy:

- Freedom: the ability of individuals (with freely chosen family or friends) to plan a life with the necessary support rather than purchase a program.
- Authority: the ability of a person with a disability (with a social support network or circle if needed) to control their own resources to purchase these supports.
- Support: How personnel and resources, formal and informal, are arranged to assist an individual with a disability to live a life in the community rich in community association and contribution.
- Responsibility: the acceptance of a valued role in a person's community through competitive employment, organizational affiliations, spiritual development, and general caring for others in the community, as well as accountability for spending public dollars in ways that are life enhancing for people with disabilities.[12]

Responsibility is beyond diversity, as it is even more embedded in organizations and human behavior. If our society can commit to these principles, people with disabilities, including those with CP, will be welcomed as part of communities and lead fulfilling lives.

To have impact on the Medicaid system, professionals need to work with their local and statewide systems and lawmakers and urge cooperation to simplify the policies and practices for people with disabilities, including those with CP, and their families.

The Plan for Inclusion[13] from UCP reports on the results of interviews conducted with key stakeholders in Florida, Maine, Michigan, New York, Texas, and Washington. These stakeholder interviews were designed to ascertain how their states achieved success in key areas, what challenges they faced, and what lessons were learned that would be helpful to all states wanting effective Medicaid services supporting full lives for individuals with intellectual and developmental disabilities. We need to outline the concrete action steps and policy initiatives from these and other research endeavors that will create change. In many cases it is not necessary to create new ways of supporting individuals, but rather to replicate the policies and strategies already proven in those states that are performing well in each area. The Plan also recommended taking action steps to promote self-direction and focus on competitive employment opportunities and strong connections to local employers. The focus needs to be on ALL people with disabilities. Services and attention have often been directed at the highest functioning individuals. The Plan advises stronger coordination between VR and competitive employment initiatives, with less operation in isolation. Beyond participation, further assessment of how many hours people with disabilities are working and for what wage is indicated, which can paint a much different picture than a simple participation measure. Other parts of the Plan emphasize self-directed, advocacy-based planning considering individual needs.[13-17]

SUMMARY

As practitioners working with young people who have moderate to severe cognitive and physical challenges, including those with cerebral palsy, the authors assert that there are best practices that make a difference. There are states and programs showing successful outcomes. Those who create partnerships among education, businesses, and rehabilitation agencies are seeing direct positive results in employment outcomes for people with disabilities, as well as cultural and perceptional changes in businesses and people who have hiring capability.

Recommendations for educators, families, and others who advocate for employment and economic independence for youth with CP include

- Be more aware of the students' abilities and assist them to reach their full potential
- Prepare them with productive and marketable skills
- Know about job options
- Have high expectations
- Plan with all community partners
- Train students for up-to-date job search skills
- Include self-determination skills in the curriculum
- Demand that technology skills are integrated into the curriculum
- Infuse the educational and avocational path with critical thinking, problem solving, teamwork, and appropriate social relationship skills
- Expect quality work
- Develop and use programs with career exploration and real-work internships immersed in business
- Expect that most youth with CP will work in a competitive, typical environment
- Put in place appropriate AT that will be used by youth with CP

- Work together to improve laws, policies, and practices toward greater diversity, welcoming people with disabilities into the workforce and every aspect of community life.
- Research practices to provide best employment and economic outcomes for youth with CP

Incremental and technical changes in our laws will not entirely fix the problems youth with CP face every day: poverty, poor educational opportunities and outcomes, little access to quality health care, high unemployment, shortages of affordable accessible housing, and limited community participation. Despite a rich and celebrated history, the disability rights movement has failed to revolutionize the public perception of disability. Expectations of employability and economic achievement must be elevated for youth with CP by themselves and their families, teachers, and caregivers. Perhaps the next great disability rights battle will be in the hearts and minds of the American public, rather than in the courts, Congress, or state capitals.[4]

REFERENCES

1. Michelsen SI, Uldall P, Kejs AM, et al. Education and employment prospects in cerebral palsy. Dev Med Child Neurol 2005;47:511–7.
2. McNaughton D, Light J, Arnold KB. Getting your wheel in the door: successful full-time employment experiences of individuals with cerebral palsy who use augmentative and alternative communication. Pennsylvania, USA: The Pennsylvania State University, University Park; 2002.
3. Liptak GS. Health and well being of adults with cerebral palsy. Curr Opin Neurol 2008;21:136–42.
4. Baker JP, Mixner DB, Harris SD. The state of disability in America: an evaluation of the disability experience by the life without limits project. Washington, DC: United Cerebral Palsy; 2009.
5. Wadsworth JS, Harper DC. The social needs of adolescents with cerebral palsy. Dev Med Child Neurol 1993;35:1019–22.
6. Stevenson CJ, Pharoah PO, Stevenson R. Cerebral palsy—the transition from youth to adulthood. Dev Med Child Neurol 1997;39:336–42.
7. Michelsen SI, Uldall P, Hansen T, et al. Social integration of adults with cerebral palsy. Dev Med Child Neurol 2006;48:643–9.
8. Murphy KP, Molnar GE, Lankasky K. Employment and social Issues in adults with cerebral palsy. Arch Phys Med Rehabil 2000;81:807–11.
9. Simon S. ADA Quarterly (Fall edition) 1998.
10. Rutkowski S, Daston M, Van Kuiken D, et al. A demand-side model of high school transition. J Vocat Rehabil 2006;25:85–96.
11. McInnes R. The power of presence: Increasing workplace receptivity. Available at: www.diversityworld.com/Disability/DN06/DN0611.htm. Accessed May 8, 2009.
12. Nerney T, Shumway D. Beyond Managed Care: Self-determination for people with disabilities. Ohio Association of County Boards of Mental Retardation and Developmental Disabilities [report]. December, 1996:3–9.
13. Bragdon T. The Plan for Inclusion, a road map for improving Medicaid for Americans with intellectual and developmental disabilities in your state [guide]. United Cerebral Palsy Organization; 2007.

14. Kaye HS. Improved employment opportunities for people with disabilities. San Francisco, CA: Disability Statistics Center, Institute for Health and Aging, University of California; May 2003.
15. Burkhauser RV, Houtenville AJ, Wittenburg D, et al. Disability Statistics. In press. Available at: www.Cornell.edu. Accessed May 8, 2009.
16. Msall ME, Rogers BT, Ripstein H, et al. Measurements of functional outcomes in children with cerebral palsy. Ment Retard Dev Disabil Res Rev 1997;3(2): 194–203.
17. Bragdon T. The Case for Inclusion 2008, UCP, Tarren Bragdon serves as Chair of the board of directors of Spurwink Services, Maine. [guide]. United Cerebral Palsy Organization; 2008.

Clinical Applications of Outcome Tools in Ambulatory Children with Cerebral Palsy

Donna J. Oeffinger, PhD[a],*, Sarah P. Rogers, MPH[b], Anita Bagley, PhD[c], George Gorton, BS[d], Chester M. Tylkowski, MD[e]

KEYWORDS

- Clinical outcomes • Cerebral palsy • Children
- Outcome tools • GMFCS

An increasing demand for evidence-based decision-making has challenged the medical community to clearly show that treatment improves a person's functional abilities within their environment. This has resulted in increased use of outcome tools in the clinical setting to supplement technical measures, such as physical examination. Outcome tools are used to measure functional performance, as a baseline descriptive assessment, to select treatment goals, and to evaluate treatment.[1] Outcome tools can help maintain patient and family motivation and provide scientific evidence on outcomes that are meaningful to patients and clinicians.

Outcome tools objectively quantify some aspect (physical, mental, or emotional) of a person. They are typically developed with a specific purpose for a target population and are used in clinical care to assess or establish treatment efficacy. They should be valid, reliable, and responsive to change. Validity is the degree to which a scale

This work was supported by Grant 9140 from the Shriners Hospitals for Children Clinical Outcomes Study Advisory Board.

[a] Pediatric Orthopedics, Shriners Hospitals for Children, 1900 Richmond Road, Lexington, KY 40502, USA

[b] Clinical Outcomes Program, Shriners Hospitals for Children, 1900 Richmond Road, Lexington, KY 40502, USA

[c] Motion Analysis Laboratory, Shriners Hospitals for Children, 2425 Stockton Boulevard, Sacramento, CA 95817, USA

[d] Clinical Outcome Assessment Laboratory, Shriners Hospitals for Children, 516 Carew Street, Springfield, MA 01104, USA

[e] Pediatric Orthopedics, Shriners Hospitals for Children, 1900 Richmond Road, Lexington, KY 40502, USA

* Corresponding author.
E-mail address: doeffinger@shrinenet.org (D.J. Oeffinger).

measures what it is intended to measure.[2] Reliability is the extent to which a measure yields consistent values over time when no change has occurred and yields consistent values between examiners.[2] Responsiveness establishes a tool's ability to detect change when a change has occurred.[3–6]

Since clinicians may lack an understanding of what to measure, lack information regarding appropriate tools, have difficulty assessing psychometric properties of tools, have doubts about clinical utility of tools, or lack the time or money for training and implementation, outcome tools are not always used by clinicians consistently, as intended, or at all.[7,8] Clinicians tend to use the easiest, most familiar, or available measure rather than what is "best" theoretically.[9]

With a goal of providing clinicians and clinician-researchers with more information on outcome tools used to assess ambulatory children with cerebral palsy (CP), this article provides an overview of several outcome tools commonly used in this population, provides research findings from a recent large multicenter study, and provides ways to integrate the research findings into clinical practice and clinical outcomes research. The information presented is the result of work conducted by the Functional Assessment Research Group (FARG), a group comprising individuals from 7 pediatric orthopedic facilities (Shriners Hospitals for Children [SHC]-Lexington, KY; SHC-Northern California; SHC-Springfield; SHC-Houston; SHC-Salt Lake City; Washington University, St. Louis; and the University of Virginia). The FARG mission is to conduct research contributing to the evidence base for treatment of the neuromusculoskeletal system in ambulatory children with CP.

In 2001, the World Health Organization (WHO) released the International Classification of Functioning, Disability and Health (ICF) framework.[10] The ICF provides a comprehensive framework to approach outcome measurement of children with disabilities.[11–13] The ICF dimensions include Body Functions and Structures, Activities and Participation, Environmental factors, and Personal factors. Health-related quality of life is not formally included in the ICF framework, but was assessed by FARG, and is defined as "what people 'feel' about their health condition or its consequences."[10]

Several outcome tools assessing the ICF dimensions of Body Functions and Structures and of Activities and Participation[14] that are frequently used in pediatric orthopedics were selected for this study. These included: the Gillette Functional Assessment Questionnaire (FAQ),[15] Gross Motor Function Measure (GMFM),[16] Pediatric Quality of Life Inventory (PedsQL),[17] Pediatric Outcomes Data Collection Instrument (PODCI),[18] Pediatric Functional Independence Measure (WeeFIM),[19] temporal-spatial gait parameters (velocity, stride length, and cadence), and energy cost during walking (O_2 cost). With the exception of FAQ Questions Two and Three and PODCI subscales of Satisfaction and Expectations, each tool has been tested for content validity and reliability.[18,20–24] These tools encompass technical measures (temporal-spatial gait parameters, O_2 cost), clinician-rated tools (GMFM D (standing) & E (walking, running, jumping), GMFM-66), parent-reported measures (WeeFIM, FAQ, PODCI, PedsQL), and child-reported measures (PODCI, PedsQL).

The Gross Motor Function Classification System (GMFCS) is a standardized classification system that categorizes the function of individuals with CP into 5 levels, with level I being the most functional and level V the least. The GMFCS is valid and reliable with excellent inter-rater reliability.[21,25–28] The FARG study focused on ambulatory children of GMFCS levels I to III: the child at level I has some motor limitations but does not use devices, at level II has limitations walking indoors and outdoors but does not use devices, and at level III has limitations walking indoors and outdoors and uses assistive devices.

GOALS OF THIS ARTICLE

The FARG study methodology, statistical analyses, and results are fully described in the series of articles published in *Developmental Medicine and Child Neurology (DMCN)*[14,29–32] and *Journal of Pediatric Orthopedics*.[33] This article will summarize the FARG study findings and succinctly answer common questions related to the clinical applications of outcome tools in children with CP. Questions related to both the cross-sectional and longitudinal study data are answered, followed by questions related to how to apply the data clinically. In addition to summarizing the study findings, examples of ways to integrate the findings into clinical practice are presented.

Cross-sectional and Longitudinal Questions

For ambulatory children with CP:

- Do outcome scores reflect differences based on GMFCS levels?
- What outcome tools best discriminate physical function?
- Do parent and child reports differ on outcome tools?
- Do children with hemiplegia function differently from those with diplegia?
- How do scores on outcome tools change over 1 year?
- Are outcome tools responsive to change?
- Does orthopedic surgery change function as measured by changes in scores on the studied outcome tools?
- What is a minimum clinically important change in outcome scores?

Clinical Practice Questions

- How do I integrate this information into my practice?
- Can I tell how the child is doing compared with others with similar severity level?
- Can I predict the normal range of scores for children with CP based on age and GMFCS level?
- How do I know if a changed score is clinically meaningful?
- Can I use outcome tools to focus on the treatment plan?

In answering these questions, comparison data are presented that will assist clinicians to understand how a child is functioning, develop individualized treatment plans, and know when a clinically meaningful change has occurred. Use of these standardized assessments can also improve communication among parents, patients, and care providers.

METHODS

This 6-year prospective multicenter study was entitled "A Cross-sectional and Longitudinal Assessment of Outcome Instruments in Patients with Ambulatory Cerebral Palsy." The study was conducted at 7 pediatric orthopedic facilities across the United States that treat children from several surrounding states. Institutional Review Board approval was obtained at each site and all participants signed consent, assent as appropriate, and privacy and confidentiality forms.

Participants

Participants were enrolled in the study which included cross-sectional and longitudinal endpoints. Inclusion criteria were: diagnosis of CP, GMFCS levels I to III, ages 4 to 18 years, and ability to complete a gait evaluation. Exclusion criteria were: previous selective dorsal rhizotomy, lower extremity orthopedic surgery within the past year, botulinum toxin-A injections within the past 6 months, or a currently operating baclofen pump.

Five hundred and sixty-two individuals completed the baseline assessments and 387 completed the follow-up evaluation (68.7%). Of those who did not complete the follow-up evaluation: 95 were unable to be contacted (16.9%), 29 declined (5.2%), 9 did not come for their follow-up appointment (1.6%), 4 were no longer ambulatory (0.7%), 2 had surgery less than 1 year from baseline to study completion (0.4%), and 36 did not participate for other reasons (6.4%). Six (1.6%) were excluded from analysis because of incomplete data, resulting in a final longitudinal sample of 381. There were no differences at baseline for age, height, weight, type of involvement, gender, GMFCS level, birth history, and ethnicity between those who completed the follow-up and those who did not.

Of the 562 participants who completed the cross-sectional component, there were 339 (60%) males, 223 (40%) females; 240 (43%) GMFCS level I, 196 (35%) Level II, and 126 (22%) Level III; 400 (71%) diplegic and 162 (29%) hemiplegic; and 83% were Caucasian. Mean age at baseline was 11.0 (standard deviation [SD] 4.3) years (range, 4.1–18.3).

For the 381 participants who completed the follow-up assessments, there were 230 (60%) males, 151 (40%) females; 174 (46%) GMFCS level I, 132 (34%) level II, and 75 (20%) level III; 265 (69%) diplegic and 116 (31%) hemiplegic; and predominately Caucasian (83%). Mean age at follow-up was 12.4 (SD 3.4) years (range, 5.2–20.5). Mean time between assessments was 1.4 (SD 0.4) years. There was no significant difference in mean age, height, weight, sex, or ethnicity distributions among GMFCS levels at either baseline or follow-up.

Between assessments, individuals received treatments based on their physician's recommendations. During the study period, 87 participants (23%) had orthopedic surgery. The remaining participants had treatments that included physical therapy, bracing, and observation.

Tools and Study Methodology

GMFM Dimensions D and E , Parent and Child PedsQL, Parent and Child PODCI, FAQ, WeeFIM, O_2 cost, temporal-spatial gait parameters, and GMFCS level were collected at baseline and follow-up done at least 1 year later. Before study initiation, consistency among coordinators was verified; local coordinators were trained in GMFCS classification, tool administration, and data collection procedures. Data were collected in a study-specific database via direct computer entry and reviewed by the project manager for completeness and accuracy. Statistical analyses performed to address each study hypothesis are described briefly in the following results sections and they were also fully described in the previously published articles.[14,29–33]

RESULTS AND CLINICAL APPLICATIONS
Do Outcome Scores Reflect Differences Based on GMFCS Level?

To gain a better understanding of the outcome tools and provide clinical comparison data on the function of individual children to their peers with CP, a descriptive analysis was completed.[14] The results showed that children in GMFCS levels I, II, and III functioned differently as measured by the study outcome tools. The mean scores for each outcome tool were clearly separated by GMFCS level. The completed results for all studied tools which included the mean, SD, range, interquartile range, and 95% confidence intervals were previously reported.[14]

Analysis of variance (ANOVA) was used to assess the relationships between outcome scores and GMFCS levels. It was determined that there were direct relationships between outcome scores and GMFCS level for Parent and Child PODCI Global Function, Transfers and Basic Mobility, Sports and Physical Function, Parent PODCI Upper Extremity and Physical Function, WeeFIM domains of Self Care and Mobility, FAQ Question One (walking scale), GMFM Dimensions D and E, GMFM-66 score, O_2 cost, and temporal-spatial gait parameters. For all of the functional assessments, as the child's severity level increased (from GMFCS I to II to III), the mean functional outcome scores decreased; an example is shown in **Fig. 1**. However, for the quality of life measures of Parent and Child PODCI Comfort/Pain, Parent and Child PODCI Happiness, Child PODCI Expectations, and Parent and Child PedsQL Emotional Functioning, children of different GMFCS levels reported a similar quality of life.

Although there was clear separation of the means, other descriptive measures of central tendency overlapped. The large sample size in this study may have contributed to finding statistically significant differences among GMFCS levels that may not have clinical significance. The ANOVA examines if the means of the groups are different and provides little information about the variation within the groups. Therefore, the degree of separation and overlap of interquartile ranges (middle half of population, 25%–75%) among GMFCS levels were reviewed. Overlap between levels shows the heterogeneous nature of CP. There was minimal overlap between the lower end of GMFCS level I scores and the upper end of level III scores. However, there was substantial overlap between the lower end of level I scores and the upper end of level II scores. These findings are consistent with the difficulties reported in classifying patients between levels I and II.[21,27] Minimal overlap was seen between the lower end of level II and the upper end of level III.

The FAQ data are nonparametric and required analyses using odds ratios. The analysis revealed that FAQ Question One showed a difference among all GMFCS levels indicating that parents' report of their child's walking ability is consistent with the clinician's gross motor rating using the GMFCS. Parents reported on FAQ Question Two what they felt limited their child's walking ability and on FAQ Question Three what skills

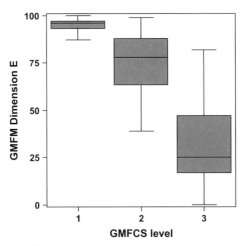

GMFCS = Gross Motor Classification System

Fig. 1. Example of clear separation of means by GMFCS level for GMFM Dimension E, GMFCS, Gross Motor Classification System.

their child is able to do under typical conditions. Only 27% of parents reported that pain limits their child's walking ability and 39% reported safety as a limiting factor. As severity level increased, a greater percentage reported safety as a problem. Regardless of GMFCS level, the majority of parents felt that balance, endurance, and weakness were limiting factors for walking. For FAQ Question Three, parents indicated that nearly all children were able to walk up and down stairs using a railing (87%), kick a ball (92%), and step over an object (90%). Only 11% of the children were able to jump rope and 15% to ice or roller skate. The parent's perspective is important to help focus goals and clinicians should be sensitive to parents' concerns when developing treatment plans.

Since the GMFCS was designed as a broad classification system based on function,[21] one would expect children in different GMFCS levels to score differently on outcome tools. The significant differences in mean outcome scores found on the tools used in this study indicate that children classified into different GMFCS levels function differently. These findings support the use of the study outcome tools to assess function and support the GMFCS as an appropriate method of classifying severity, despite some overlap between levels. Examples of the differences among GMFCS levels for the studied outcome tools are reported in **Table 1**.

What Outcome Tools Best Discriminate Physical Function in Ambulatory Children with CP?

Knowing which tools best discriminate among GMFCS levels can assist in the selection of tools for clinical or research use, since it is not practical and often not feasible to administer multiple tools during a single visit.[29] The best outcome tool, however, is dependent upon the clinical/research question and clinical/research endpoints of interest. The recommendations presented here focus on the tools assessed in this study that were the most discriminatory among GMFCS levels.

Using effect size indices (ESIs) for parametric variables and odds ratios for nonparametric data, the magnitude of differences in scores on the study tools across GMFCS levels were quantified. Binary logistic regression models determined discrimination, and receiver operating characteristic (ROC) curves addressed sensitivity and specificity of the measures.

Based on the study tools' ability to discriminate (large ESIs) among GMFCS levels, the best tools to measure physical function in ambulatory children with CP are the GMFM Dimension E or GMFM-66, the Parent report PODCI Sports and Physical Function, Global Function, and the FAQ Question One. Tools that performed well and that are good secondary measures are the WeeFIM Self Care and Mobility domains and temporal-spatial gait parameters. The least discriminatory tools were the quality of life and cognition measures; however, these are important in comprehensive assessments of treatment effects.

Table 1
Example of select outcome tool means and SDs by GMFCS level

Outcome Tool	GMFCS I Mean (SD)	GMFCS II Mean (SD)	GMFCS III Mean (SD)
GMFM D- standing	94 (6)	84 (8)	52 (24)
GMFM E- walking	93 (8)	75 (16)	32 (20)
Energy (O_2) cost (mL O_2/kg/m)	0.28 (0.1)	0.38 (0.2)	0.57 (0.3)
Parent PODCI global function	81 (11)	72 (12)	62 (13)
Parent PODCI sports	68 (17)	51 (17)	35 (17)

ROC curves were constructed to determine sensitivity and specificity for the most discriminant measures identified by regression models. Based on this analysis, the single most discriminatory measure of physical function, as classified by the GMFCS, is the GMFM-66 score. This is the Rasch-analyzed score of the GMFM using the Gross Motor Activity Estimator program. Rasch analysis equalizes the difference between points on the scale, creating an interval scale, such that the interval of change from 15 to 25 is equivalent to the change from 65 to 75. The GMFM-66 is the best clinical choice for discriminating among GMFCS levels I through III.

A tool's discriminatory ability may be limited by ceiling effects. Ceiling effects suggest that either the participants do not have significant limitations in these areas, or that there is a need for more challenging "upper end" items or questions. Parent and Child reports of PODCI Comfort/Pain and WeeFIM Cognition have large ceiling effects for all three GMFCS levels, suggesting that pain and limitations in cognition are not major issues for these children or that the questions are too easy to identify if such issues are present.

As an example of a tool with limited discriminatory ability, **Fig. 2** shows a box plot of the Parent report of PODCI Comfort/Pain scores. Note that there are no upper fences for any GMFCS level, showing ceiling effects. The boxes represent the interquartile ranges for the data, presenting the range of scores obtained by the middle 50% of the participants for each GMFCS level. The size of the boxes shows variability within GMFCS level and degree of overlap between GMFCS levels. For the example shown, ceiling effects and the overlap of interquartile ranges limit the discriminatory ability of this subscale.

Do Parent and Child Reports Differ on Outcome Tools?

The PODCI and PedsQL have parent and child report forms. Given the time constraints often present in the clinical setting, it would helpful to know if completion by both parent and child are necessary. Therefore, differences in parent and child responses on the same tools were studied.[14] A direct relationship (as severity increased scores decreased) between outcome scores and GMFCS levels was

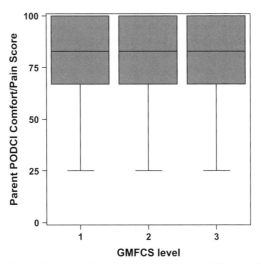

Fig. 2. Example of ceiling effects and limited discriminatory ability in all GMFCS levels for Parent PODCI Comfort/Pain score.

seen for both the parent and child reports, despite the differences noted between scores. For 2 of the tools studied, the PODCI and PedsQL, there are both a parent and child report version. Results showed that there were differences between the scores reported by the parent and the child. Children scored themselves higher than their parents for almost all PODCI and PedsQL subscales.[14] As the child's GMFCS level increased, the differences between parent and child scores increased. Physical subscales of PODCI Sports and Physical Function and PedsQL Physical Functioning showed the greatest differences. Example data are presented in **Table 2**.

This is not the case for able-bodied children, who tend to report the same scores as their parents.[34,35] The authors speculate that these findings are likely related to perspectives of disability. The child's perception is one of ability, since the impairment was not acquired after a period of normal development. The child emphasizes what he can do. Parents have the expectation that their child should be able to do everything able-bodied children can. Therefore, the parent's perspective is more likely one of disability and emphasizes what the child cannot do. For these reasons, it is important to obtain both parent and child perspectives on goals and outcomes.

Do Children with Hemiplegia Differ from Children with Diplegia?

Children with hemiplegia compared with those with diplegia were assessed, since grouping of children with CP with notably different clinical presentations, and presumably different profiles of brain injury, may lead to inaccurate predictions of developmental rate and prognosis.[30]

Based on the scores of the studied outcome tools, children with hemiplegia function differently from those with diplegia. Differences in outcome scores between these groups within GMFCS levels were tested and children with hemiplegia consistently scored lower on tools related to upper extremity and school function, and higher on nearly all tools that assessed gait or lower extremity function.[30]

Ceiling effects were shown to be a function of the diagnostic subtype, GMFCS level, and outcome tool. They were mostly higher in GMFCS level I. The ceiling effects reflected the different strengths in each of the groups and were not consistently higher in either diagnostic subtype. For example, the children with hemiplegia had a higher percentage of ceiling effects in the PODCI Transfers and Basic Mobility subscale and WeeFIM Mobility, which shows their reliably higher scores on lower extremity functional assessments. However, the children with diplegia had a higher percentage of ceiling effects on WeeFIM Self Care, which shows their somewhat better upper extremity function. It is important to note that these ceiling effects may have made differences between diagnostic subtypes less evident.

Objective evidence of the distinct differences between children with diplegia and hemiplegia within the same GMFCS classification level exists in various aspects of motor functioning, activity, participation, and quality of life. Using GMFCS level alone

Table 2		
Example of difference in Parent versus Child report for select PODCI and PedsQL subscales		
Outcome Tool	**Parent Mean (SD)**	**Child Mean (SD)**
PODCI sports	57 (21)	70 (19)
PODCI upper extremity	84 (14)	93 (10)
PODCI transfers	86 (13)	93 (9)
PedsQL physical functioning	57 (19)	69 (19)
PedsQL social functioning	57 (19)	65 (22)

as a predictor of motor prognosis may overestimate the lower extremity skills of children with diplegia, and underestimate those of children with hemiplegia.

How Do Scores Change on Outcome Tools for Ambulatory Children with CP Over 1 Year?

Since children with chronic conditions such as CP are assessed repeatedly over time, it is important to know the expected amount of change as a result of natural history.[31] Expected changes can be used by clinicians to assess whether observed changes with time are atypical, thus influencing treatment planning. Change data on the 381 individuals who completed both the baseline and follow-up assessments were analyzed. For the studied tools, small mean changes with large SDs were seen over a 1-year period. The small mean changes were a result of the outcome tool change scores being normally distributed, with some large positive and negative changes. The large variability in change scores is likely because of the heterogeneity of CP. Complete results were published by Oeffinger and colleagues[31] in 2008; sample results are presented in **Table 3**. In addition, the average change scores and SDs are presented by GMFCS level and surgical or nonsurgical group by Oeffinger and colleagues[31] (2008). Since changes that occur over a year are often small, one should be particularly cognizant of those individuals that present with large changes in function in a short period of time.

Are Outcome Tools Responsive to Change?

Analyses were completed to determine if the tools were responsive to change despite small mean changes over a 1-year period.[31] To assess the responsiveness of the tools, a known change in function was needed. The investigators used a verified change in GMFCS level between assessments as a known change in function. Based on the analysis, the outcome tools were responsive when a change in function occurred large enough to result in a change in GMFCS level. The tools that were the most responsive to change were the functional subscales (GMFM Dimensions D and E; GMFM-66; Parent PODCI, Global Function, Transfers and Sports; gait velocity; and stride length). Large changes in function were reflected appropriately on the outcome tools. As function improved, the outcome scores increased and as function decreased, the outcome scores decreased. Additional research must be conducted to determine the most responsive tools, which can vary based upon GMFCS level and endpoints of interest.

Table 3			
Example of mean change scores and SDs for select outcome tools by GMFCS level			
Outcome Tool	**GMFCS I Mean (SD)**	**GMFCS II Mean (SD)**	**GMFCS III Mean (SD)**
GMFM-66	0.2 (5.4)	0.8 (3.5)	0.5 (3.5)
Velocity (% normal)	−0.8 (16.5)	0.5 (16.2)	−0.9 (15.2)
Parent PODCI sports	1.0 (12.4)	2.5 (13.9)	2.1 (13.2)
Parent PODCI upper extremity	3.9 (10.0)	3.9 (11.6)	1.6 (9.8)
Parent PedsQL transfers	0.6 (10.8)	2.5 (10.3)	2.3 (12.1)
Parent PedsQL physical	−0.4 (16.5)	1.8 (16.9)	−0.7 (18.9)
Parent PedsQL social functioning	2.4 (15.8)	4.1 (17.3)	3.8 (15.2)
WeeFIM mobility	−0.1 (4.2)	0.7 (8.2)	0.8 (8.8)
WeeFIM self care	0.8 (7.3)	2.0 (11.0)	3.0 (10.4)

Does Orthopedic Surgery Change Function as Measured by Changes in Scores on the Studied Outcome Measures?

Lower extremity musculotendinous surgery is a standard treatment for ambulatory children with CP who have joint contractures and bony torsions.[36] Ultimately, the objectives of surgical management in CP are to improve function, decrease discomfort, and prevent disabling structural changes.[37,38] The assumption is that by improving gait, function in general will improve. Therefore, data from a subset of 75 individuals who underwent lower extremity surgery were evaluated and their changes compared with changes in a matched nonsurgical group.[36]

The 75 participants who had surgery during the study period were individually matched with 1 of the 294 participants who did not have surgery. For each surgical participant, all nonsurgical participants who exactly matched by gender, GMFCS level and type of involvement (hemiplegic or diplegic) were identified. The surgical procedures included both soft tissue and bone surgery. The nonsurgical group had a standard of care treatment within the study window. This included observation, stretching and strengthening exercises, bracing, and medication management, if necessary.

The mean change scores showed that lower extremity orthopedic surgery is effective in improving gait, but these improvements do not necessarily translate into large changes in outcome tool scores. The greatest changes as a result of lower extremity surgical intervention occurred at the ICF Body Structure and Function level, closest to the level of surgical intervention. The FARG study found that surgery significantly improves gait kinematics as measured by the Gillette Gait Index (GGI), which quantifies the magnitude of deviation from normal gait. The greater the severity level, the greater the magnitude of change in GGI from pre- to postoperative. However, the improvements in gait did not translate into significant changes in measures of Activity and Participation. These data suggest that the outcome tools are not sufficiently responsive to measure the effect gait improvements have on Activity and Participation, or that there are no such changes. The complete analysis and findings are in press (Gorton and colleagues[36]).

What is a Minimum Clinically Important Difference in Changes in Outcome Scores?

Although statistically significant differences are important, it is more relevant for evidence-based practice to define clinically significant changes.[31] Reported changes frequently reach statistical significance, but may not be clinically meaningful.[39,40] Clinically meaningful infers different connotations to the child, family, and clinician. Minimum clinically important differences (MCIDs) are often subjectively defined, based on training and experience. MCIDs can also be quantified objectively and have been defined and calculated in various ways.[16,35,41–43] In this study, MCID is defined as the magnitude of change required for an observable difference in function, and it is quantified using effect sizes. Effect size is a unitless measurement of the number of SDs from the mean (mean/SD). Small effect sizes may be described as imperceptible to the human eye, medium as large enough to be seen in normal observation, and large as grossly observable.[6]

MCIDs were calculated using the data from the longitudinal component of the study. The details of the analysis were reported by Oeffinger and colleagues[31] (2008). MCIDs were established for the GMFM, PODCI, PedsQL, WeeFIM, O_2 cost, and temporal-spatial gait parameters for ambulatory children with CP. Change scores exceeding MCIDs for medium effect sizes are considered large enough to be clinically meaningful. Sample results from data previously reported in *DMCN*[31] are shown in **Table 4**.

Table 4
Example of minimum clinically important difference (MCID) scores for medium (0.5)
and large (0.8) effect sizes on select outcome tools

Outcome Tool	GMFCS Level I MCID Medium (0.5)	GMFCS Level I MCID Large (0.8)	GMFCS Level II MCID Medium (0.5)	GMFCS Level II MCID Large (0.8)	GMFCS Level III MCID Medium (0.5)	GMFCS Level III MCID Large (0.8)	Combined GMFCS I–III MCID Medium (0.5)	Combined GMFCS I–III MCID Large (0.8)
GMFM-66	1.7	2.7	1	1.5	0.7	1.2	0.8	1.3
O_2 cost (mL O_2/kg/min)	0.04	0.06	0.11	0.17	0.06	0.09	0.06	0.09
Velocity (% normal)	8.7	13.9	6.8	10.9	5.5	8.8	5.7	9.1
Parent PODCI global function	4.5	7.2	4.9	7.9	2.8	4.5	3.8	6
Parent PODCI sports	4.6	7.3	6	9.7	5.7	9	4.3	6.8
Parent PedsQL school	7.1	11.4	8.6	13.8	7.7	12.3	7.7	12.3

TRANSLATION INTO CLINICAL PRACTICE

When data from studies are reported in the literature, the next critical step is the translation of this knowledge into information to help clinicians understand how to use the data in their daily clinical practice.

How Do I Integrate this Information into My Clinical Practice?

Identify outcomes of importance and relevance to your practice. Select tools to match your focus and to best answer your clinical or research questions.[14,29–33,36] Each measure has unique characteristics and examines different parameters. For example, there are measures that quantify physical function, activity, participation, quality of life, or a combination. Similarly, there are tools designed to capture parent report, child report, or clinician ratings. The limitations of each measure must be understood, including ceiling effects, parent versus child report, and whether the population is hemiplegic versus diplegic. Once tools have been selected, you can develop a protocol for administering them routinely in your practice and using the resulting data for evaluation, treatment planning, and outcomes assessment.

Can You Tell How the Child is Doing Compared to Others of Similar Severity Level?

Clinicians should compare the child's score to the descriptive data presented for ambulatory children with CP by GMFCS level, age, and diagnostic subtype when possible.[14,31] The descriptive data include means, SDs, 95% confidence intervals, and interquartile ranges for each tool assessed.

By comparing the child's score to the mean and interquartile range, you can determine the child's ability relative to average for their peers. For example, if the child's score falls below the interquartile range, the child is doing worse than 75% of his peers. You can then assess reasons why the child may be performing poorly and focus the rehabilitation or therapy interventions on those areas. Similarly, if the score is above the interquartile range, the child is performing better than 75% of her peers and interventions may not be needed.

Can I Predict What the Normal Range of Scores is for a Child with CP Based on Age and GMFCS Level?

For the Parent report of PODCI, prediction equations have been developed for each of the subscales based on age and GMFCS level.[33] The prediction equations provide expected scores for a child, depending on age and GFMCS level, along with a range in which the predicted score may reside. Formulas exist for the following PODCI subscales: Upper Extremity Function; Transfers and Basic Mobility; Sports and Physical Function; Comfort/Pain; Global Function (composite of the 4 functional assessments); and Happiness.

Using the formulas and substituting for an individual child's age and GMFCS level, the evaluating clinician can predict the score the child should have on the particular PODCI subscale. By comparing the child's actual score to the predicted score, clinicians can determine how the child is doing compared with his or her peers with CP.

Below is an example of how to calculate the expected score for the Parent report of PODCI Transfers and Basic Mobility for an 11 year + 3-months old patient with CP in GMFCS level I using the appropriate formula.

Formula:

$$\text{Predicted transfers score} = 78.375 + (\text{age} \times 1.069 - G2 \times 8.460 - G3 \times 26.037)$$

Age, actual age in years with decimal fraction; $G2$, GMFCS level II ($0 = $ no, $1 = $ yes); $G3$, GMFCS level III ($0 = $ no, $1 = $ yes). GMFCS level I is the default for the equations.
Formula with substitutions appropriate to the example above:

$$\text{Predicted transfers} = 78.375 + (11.25 \times 1.069 - 0 \times 8.460 - 0 \times 26.037)$$

Predicted Transfers Score $= 90.401$ with a SEE of ± 11.9

SEE indicates standard error of the estimate and is a constant specific to each PODCI dimension.

The patient's actual score for this visit was 85. While the patient scored a little less than the expected score of 90, she is still well within the expected range (78–100). Treatment goals may include maintaining function in this area. One can determine areas of focus for treatment by examining the individual questions that make up the summary subscale. For example, questions that are part of the Transfer and Mobility subscale include "During the last week was it easy or hard for your child to: Climb one flight of stairs? Get on and off a toilet or chair? Sit in a regular chair without holding on?" If the patient scores at or above the expected score, appropriate treatment planning would be to maintain or possibly increase function, depending on the patient, family, and clinician goals. Alternatively, the family and clinician may choose to focus the treatment plan on areas in which the child is less functional in comparison to peers, as determined by the outcome scores.

How Do I Know if a Change Score is Clinically Meaningful?

By using the same outcome tools over time, you can determine if the child is improving or declining by comparing his or her score changes to expected changes of peers in the same GMFCS level.[31] As previously seen, MCIDs were defined for all of the studied outcome tools and reported by Oeffinger and colleagues.[31] These MCIDs can be used as guidelines for the amount of change that is clinically important. However, because of the methods used to calculate the MCIDs, they are most appropriately applied to changes in groups or between groups. This can be particularly useful for researchers when trying to determine if a statistical difference is clinically meaningful. On the individual level, it is important to ask the child's and family's opinions related to the change in function when changes in outcome scores are measured.

As established by Oeffinger and colleagues,[31] MCID is change that exceeds the value required for a medium effect size. If changes in a group's outcome tool scores exceed the reported MCID values, a change beyond natural progression is likely to have occurred. If the difference between groups is larger than the MCID threshold, the difference between groups is clinically significant. MCID thresholds can assist clinicians and researchers in advancing interpretations from being based strictly on statistical significance or subjective clinical judgment, to being based on consistent quantitative evidence.

For example, a group of individuals with CP (GMFCS levels I–III) participated in a research study that examined function using velocity (% normal) before and after botulinum toxin-A injections. To reach a MCID at a medium effect size, a change of 5.7% between assessments is needed, and a change of 9.1% is needed to reach a large effect size. The mean at baseline was 75% and at 3-months post-injection was 82%. There was an improvement of 7% which was statistically different and also clinically significant since the change exceeded the MCID for a medium effect size.

Can I Use Outcome Tools to Focus the Treatment Plan?

The findings of the FARG study can be used in developing the treatment plan and goals.[14,29–33,36] Based on the information provided in this article and the data presented in the study publications, you can objectively assess a child's current functional level and use the scores to focus areas of treatment, thus saving time and improving the cost-effectiveness of your practice. You can then objectively reassess the child's function over time to determine if a significant change has taken place and adjust treatment prescriptions and goals accordingly.

GENERALIZABILITY AND LIMITATIONS

These findings are appropriate to generalize for children with CP in GMFCS levels I to III and between the ages of 4 and 18 years. Since the majority of the study population was Caucasian (83%) and were English speaking, the study findings may have limited applicability to minority or non-English speaking children with CP.

Several challenges exist with administration of outcome tools in the clinical environment. First, there are a limited number of validated tools available to clinicians that have been studied and have comparison data available for use. Also, implementing a process for routine use of outcome tools that is accepted by staff can be met with resistance. If you are successful in implementing a process, long-term commitment to the process in the clinical setting can be difficult because of limits in clinical resources such as time, personnel, costs associated with purchasing and licensing, and fees for the outcome tools. Inefficient methods for data management and poor accessibility to data lead to little or no use of the collected information. Difficulties can exist in finding accessible comparison data in user-friendly formats for normal and diagnosis-specific populations.

These challenges can be overcome through education of clinicians regarding the usefulness and importance of outcome assessments. Selection of optimal outcome tools that provide meaningful information for all those involved and that can be completed in a timely manner are critical first steps to a successful outcomes improvement program. Establishing protocols for administration and review of the data collected from the outcome tools, along with a method to assure follow-through with the established protocols, is necessary for success. Implementing changes in practice is difficult, but the difficulty can be overcome more quickly if training and coaching are provided by advanced clinicians, real-time outcomes feedback is provided to the clinician and patient, and synthesized research evidence is easily available at the point of care.[8,44] Electronic information systems, such as databases, can provide real-time feedback; synthesized comparative research evidence at the point of care; and reduce time burdens for patients, families, and clinicians for data collection and comparison purposes. These suggestions must be tailored to your specific facility, where a multifaceted approach to clinician behavior change must address various local barriers and must engage clinicians.[45] A successfully implemented outcomes improvement program balances the thoroughness of the clinical assessment with the burdens on the patient and family to complete the outcome tools and on the clinician to obtain the results. The outcomes assessed should be meaningful to clinicians and patients and lead to improved evidence-based practice.

SUMMARY

The summary presented here and in the referenced articles provides information on: outcome tools' discriminatory ability and responsiveness; readily available comparison data on 7 commonly used outcome measures that can be used at the point of care for ambulatory children with CP; prediction equations for the Parent report PODCI by age and GMFCS level; and minimum clinically important difference thresholds by GMFCS level. This information can assist the clinician in selecting the best tools to discriminate among levels of severity and avoid ceiling effects. By documenting the results of care, you can provide objective assessment of changes from pretreatment status and monitor progress toward achievement of treatment goals, which helps to maintain patient motivation. It helps the clinician to know when to adjust or discontinue a program and can also help justify reimbursement.

When using the data presented to compare a child's score to a population score, outlier scores become evident and may trigger patient reassessment to determine potential causes and courses of action. The scores allow direct comparisons between a specific patient and a matched cohort, assisting clinicians in the creation of comprehensive and individualized management plans. Understanding functional levels of an individual child with CP relative to other children with CP, before and after operative and nonoperative interventions, potentially provides insights into the benefits of specific treatment modalities. Outcome tools should be used in the clinical assessment of children with CP to assess outcomes that are meaningful to patients and families, document results of care, detect an indication for treatment, aid in treatment choice, and evaluate treatments to determine if the goals were met. Use of appropriate outcome tools can lead to best practices and reduced costs in the clinical setting.

ACKNOWLEDGMENTS

This work was funded by Shriners Hospitals for Children (SHC), Clinical Outcomes Study Advisory Board Grant # 9140, "A Cross-sectional and Longitudinal Assessment of Outcome Instruments in Patients with Ambulatory Cerebral Palsy." The authors acknowledge the participation of the Functional Assessment Research Group study investigators (Mark Abel, MD, and Mark Romness, MD, University of Virginia; Doug Barnes, MD, Elroy Sullivan, PhD, and Judi Linton, BS, SHC-Houston;

Diane Damiano, PhD, Washington University; Diane Nicholson, PhD, SHC-Salt Lake City) and coordinators from each site. The authors would also like to acknowledge the patients and their families for their participation.

REFERENCES

1. Ottenbacher KJ, Msall ME, Lyon NR, et al. Interrater agreement and stability of the Functional Independence Measure for children (WeeFIM): use in children with developmental disabilities. Arch Phys Med Rehabil 1997;78(B):1309–15.
2. Portney L, Watkins M. Foundations of clinical research: applications to practice. 3rd edition. Upper Saddle River (NJ): Prentice Hall; 2008.
3. De Bruin AF, Diederiks JP, De Witte LP, et al. Assessing the responsiveness of a functional status measure: the sickness impact profile versus the SIP68. J Clin Epidemiol 1997;50(B):529–40.
4. Garratt A, Hutchinson A, Russell I, Network for Evidence-Based Practice in Northern and Yorkshire (NEBPINY). The UK version of the Seattle Angina Questionnaire (SAQ-UK): reliability, validity and responsiveness. J Clin Epidemiol 2001;54(B):907–15.
5. Kirshner B, Guyatt G. A methodological framework for assessing health indices. J Chronic Dis 1985;38:27–36.
6. Portney L, Watkins MP. Foundations of clinical research: applications to practice. 2nd edition. Upper Saddle River (NJ): Prentice Hall Health; 2000.
7. Grimshaw J. Changing physicians' behavior: what works and thoughts on getting more things to work. J Contin Educ Health Prof 2002;22:237–43.
8. Haynes B. Barriers and bridges to evidence based clinical practice. BMJ 1998; 317:273–6.
9. Ketelaar M, Vermeer A, Helders PJ. Functional motor abilities of children with cerebral palsy: a systematic literature review of assessment measures. Clin Rehabil 1998;12(A):369–80.
10. WHO. ICF: International classification of functioning, disability and health. Geneva: World Health Organization; 2001.
11. Beckung E, Hagberg G. Correlation between ICIDH handicap code and gross motor function classification system in children with cerebral palsy. Dev Med Child Neurol 2000;42(B):669–73.
12. Majnemer A, Mazer B. New directions in the outcome evaluation of children with cerebral palsy. Semin Pediatr Neurol 2004;11:11–7.
13. Ostensjo S, Carlberg EB, Vollestad NK. Everyday functioning in young children with cerebral palsy: functional skills, caregiver assistance, and modifications of the environment. Dev Med Child Neurol 2003;45(B):603–12.
14. Oeffinger D, Gorton G, Bagley A, et al. Outcome assessments in children with cerebral palsy, part I: descriptive characteristics of GMFCS Levels I to III. Dev Med Child Neurol 2007;49(B):172–80.
15. Novacheck TF, Stout JL, Tervo R. Reliability and validity of the Gillette Functional Assessment Questionnaire as an outcome measure in children with walking disabilities. J Pediatr Orthop 2000;20(B):75–81.
16. Russell DJ, Rosenbaum PL, Avery LM, Lane M. Gross motor function measure (GMFM-66 & GMFM-88) user's manual. Hamilton, Ontario: Mac Keith Press; 2002.
17. Varni JW, Seid M, Rode CA. The PedsQL: measurement model for the pediatric quality of life inventory. Med Care 1999;37(B):126–39.
18. Daltroy LH, Liang MH, Fossel AH, et al. The POSNA pediatric musculoskeletal functional health questionnaire: report on reliability, validity, and sensitivity to

change. Pediatric Outcomes Instrument Development Group. Pediatric Orthopaedic Society of North America. J Pediatr Orthop 1998;18(B):561–71.

19. McCabe MA, Granger CV. Content validity of a pediatric functional independence measure. Appl Nurs Res 1990;3(B):120–2.

20. Nordmark E, Hagglund G, Jarnlo GB. Reliability of the gross motor function measure in cerebral palsy. Scand J Rehabil Med 1997;29(B):25–8.

21. Palisano R, Rosenbaum P, Walter S, et al. Development and reliability of a system to classify gross motor function in children with cerebral palsy. Dev Med Child Neurol 1997;39(B):214–23.

22. Russell DJ, Avery LM, Rosenbaum PL, et al. Improved scaling of the gross motor function measure for children with cerebral palsy: evidence of reliability and validity. Phys Ther 2000;80(B):873–85.

23. Varni JW, Seid M, Kurtin PS. PedsQL 4.0: reliability and validity of the pediatric quality of life inventory version 4.0 generic core scales in healthy and patient populations. Med Care 2001;39(B):800–12.

24. Wong V, Wong S, Chan K, et al. Functional Independence Measure (WeeFIM) for Chinese children: Hong Kong cohort. Pediatrics 2002 Feb;109(2):317–9.

25. Morris C, Bartlett D. Gross motor function classification system: impact and utility. Dev Med Child Neurol 2004;46(B):60–5.

26. Oeffinger DJ, Tylkowski CM, Rayens MK, et al. Gross motor function classification system and outcome tools for assessing ambulatory cerebral palsy: a multicenter study. Dev Med Child Neurol 2004;46(B):311–9.

27. Palisano RJ, Hanna SE, Rosenbaum PL, et al. Validation of a model of gross motor function for children with cerebral palsy. Phys Ther 2000;80:974–85.

28. Rosenbaum PL. Prognosis for gross motor development in cerebral palsy. Creation of motor growth curves. JAMA 2002;288(B):1357–63.

29. Bagley AM, Gorton G, Oeffinger D, et al. Outcome assessments in children with cerebral palsy, part II: discriminatory ability of outcome tools. Dev Med Child Neurol 2007;49(B):181–6.

30. Damiano D, Abel M, Romness M, et al. Comparing functional profiles of children with hemiplegic and diplegic cerebral palsy in GMFCS Levels I and II: are separate classifications needed? Dev Med Child Neurol 2006;48(B):797–803.

31. Oeffinger D, Bagley A, Rogers S, et al. Outcome tools used for ambulatory children with cerebral palsy: responsiveness and minimum clinically important differences. Dev Med Child Neurol 2008;50(B):918–25.

32. Sullivan E, Barnes D, Linton JL, et al. Relationships among functional outcome measures used for assessing children with ambulatory CP. Dev Med Child Neurol 2007;49(B):338–44.

33. Barnes D, Linton JL, Sullivan E, et al. Pediatric outcomes data collection instrument scores in ambulatory children with cerebral palsy: an analysis by age groups and severity level. J Pediatr Orthop 2008;28(B):97–102.

34. Haynes RJ, Sullivan E. The Pediatric Orthopaedic Society of North America pediatric orthopaedic functional health questionnaire: an analysis of normals. J Pediatr Orthop 2001;21(B):619–21.

35. Varni JW, Burwinkle TM, Jacobs JR, et al. The PedsQL in type 1 and type 2 diabetes: reliability and validity of the pediatric quality of life inventory generic core scales and type 1 diabetes module. Diabetes Care 2003;26(B):631–7.

36. Gorton G, Abel M, Oeffinger D, et al. What are the effects of lower extremity orthopedic surgery on outcome measures in ambulatory children with cerebral palsy? J Pediat Orthop 2009, submitted for publication.

37. Karol LA. Surgical management of the lower extremity in ambulatory children with cerebral palsy. J Am Acad Orthop Surg 2004;12:196–203.
38. Sprague JB. Surgical management of cerebral palsy. Orthop Nurs 1992;11:11–9.
39. Carney BT, Oeffinger D, Gove NK. Sagittal knee kinematics after rectus femoris transfer without hamstring lengthening. J Pediatr Orthop 2006;26(B):265–70.
40. Gage JR, Fabian D, Hicks R, et al. Pre- and postoperative gait analysis in patients with spastic diplegia: a preliminary report. J Pediatr Orthop 1984;4(B):715–25.
41. Bowen TR, Lennon N, Castagno P, et al. Variability of energy-consumption measures in children with cerebral palsy. J Pediatr Orthop 1998;18(B):738–42.
42. Ottenbacher KJ, Msall ME, Lyon N, et al. The WeeFIM instrument: its utility in detecting change in children with developmental disabilities. Arch Phys Med Rehabil 2000;81(B):1317–26.
43. Wang HH, Liao HF, Hsieh CL. Reliability, sensitivity to change, and responsiveness of the peabody developmental motor scales-second edition for children with cerebral palsy. Phys Ther 2006;86(B):51–6.
44. Doran DM, Sidani S. Outcomes-focused knowledge translation: a framework for knowledge translation and patient outcomes improvement. Worldviews Evid Based Nurs 2007;4:3–13.
45. Grimshaw J. Changing provider behavior–an overview of systematic reviews of interventions (part 3). Med Care 2001;39(A)(II):2–45.

Understanding Function and Other Outcomes in Cerebral Palsy

Jilda Vargus-Adams, MD, MSc[a,b,*]

KEYWORDS

- Cerebral palsy • Outcome • Clinical trials
- Function • Disability

Care and research in childhood cerebral palsy (CP) is evolving. The process of change requires careful attention to understanding the status of children with CP—how and what they are doing, the things that are challenging, and the ways in which they adapt to their challenges. Outcome measurement is the way in which the status of patients and research subjects is described. Outcomes are any of the things that can be measured and encompass all parameters of human existence, from blood tests to walking speed to quality of life. The tools used to measure outcomes may be laboratory tests, physical examinations, questionnaires, interviews, or any other evaluations. These tools may be called outcome measures, instruments, or assessments. In CP, outcome measurement is a prominent and important topic, especially because having robust means of measuring outcomes is vital to understanding the usefulness of treatments. If research cannot accurately measure the things that matter for children with CP, then it cannot establish if interventions are having useful effects. This article addresses the challenges of outcome measurement in CP, the current status of outcome measurement in CP, and the issues of understanding change in childhood CP.

MEASUREMENT CHALLENGES WITH CEREBRAL PALSY

The measurement of outcomes in children with cerebral palsy presents an array of challenges. The issues of concern for children with CP are wide-ranging, chronic,

This work has been supported by National Institutes of Health Child Health and Human Development K23 HD049552 and United Cerebral Palsy Research and Education Foundation EH-008-06.
[a] Division of Pediatric Rehabilitation, Departments of Pediatrics and Physical Medicine & Rehabilitation, Cincinnati Children's Hospital Medical Center, University of Cincinnati College of Medicine, 3333 Burnet Avenue, MLC 4009, Cincinnati, Ohio 45229-3039, USA
[b] Center for Epidemiology and Biostatistics, Cincinnati Children's Hospital Medical Center, University of Cincinnati College of Medicine, 3333 Burnet Avenue, MLC 4009, Cincinnati, Ohio 45229-3039, USA
* Corresponding author.
E-mail address: jilda.vargus-adams@cchmc.org

difficult to quantify, resistant to change, and more reflective of disability than illness. These parameters lead to frustration for the clinician or researcher who wishes to evaluate the status of a child or youth with CP.

CP impacts a breadth of arenas. Any person with CP, parent, or medical professional who cares for children with CP will attest that CP touches almost every aspect of life. CP causes changes in basic body functioning, such as strength, coordination, and muscle tone. CP results in difficulty with functional tasks, such as walking, swallowing, accomplishing self-care, and communicating. In turn, these deficits contribute to decreased involvement in community, school, and family activities. CP has some impact on quality of life[1] and definitely creates additional stressors for caregivers.[2] These facts illustrate the many potential problem areas to understand and to measure in CP. The sheer number of possible targets for measurement makes it hard to describe CP in a comprehensive and accurate fashion.

CP is a diverse diagnosis with substantial variation in impairments and severity. Although CP may manifest with marked impairments and myriad secondary impacts, some individuals with CP have fairly modest disability and few daily effects. CP is highly associated with other conditions, including cognitive impairment and epilepsy, that create their own issues. Because of the variability in symptoms, sequelae, and co-morbidities, any 2 children with CP may look very different from each other. Understanding how those 2 different children are doing may mean using 2 entirely different evaluations that are targeted to the issues affecting each child. These differences create a need for flexibility in measurement strategies so as to address each child with CP in a meaningful way.

Another challenge is the long-term nature of CP. CP is not an acute illness. Children and youth with CP will always have CP, but their CP may affect them differently over time. It is of paramount importance to understand the long-term outcomes of CP and how interventions affect outcomes many years later. Studying outcomes in a longitudinal fashion for years, rather than weeks or months, is expensive, time-consuming, and messy because of the inability to control for extraneous factors. Nonetheless, longitudinal measurement is arguably the most important method to explore treatments and interventions for CP, as outcomes in adolescence and adulthood are of critical importance.

There are few gold standards or rubrics for measurement in CP. Many of the domains of concern are not easily quantified, and there are no established benchmarks of measurement. For example, there is no single, best, and universally accepted method to measure even how well a child with CP walks. Assessing things such as quality of movement, happiness, ease of care, and independence is a confusing and frustrating venture. Unlike more quantifiable outcomes (eg, blood pressure or birth weight), most concerns in CP do not have an established "ruler" to measure them.

One goal of outcome measurement is to assess changes that occur as a result of treatments or interventions. This is another concern in CP because so many of the available treatments do not seem to create big changes. With small treatment effects described for many interventions, at least with the available measurement tools, a question arises: Are the available outcome measures really good enough? Either the measurement tools are not adequately sensitive to change and cannot detect meaningful effects of treatment or the treatments have insufficient effect to be meritorious. Until each individual outcome measure can be evaluated for its discriminatory properties and responsiveness to change, this conundrum will remain.

A final challenge in measurement in CP is the difficulty of looking at CP with a purely medical perspective. This perspective considers CP to be a disease and people with

CP to be ill. It suggests that CP is something that has clear biologic markers and that medical interventions can or should be used to alter the underlying disease process. These ideas translate into a measurement paradigm that includes an assumption that the basic processes of CP should be targeted with treatments and that improving the physiologic parameters of CP will result in improvements in the outcomes of interest. This is how things work for most health conditions. In the case of CP, however, this approach is not entirely satisfactory. First of all, many people with CP are not ill and are best described as having a disability rather than poor health. When viewed as a chronic disability, CP is not something that is readily amenable to direct treatment. Furthermore, the degree of impairment in the more "basic" issues of CP (eg, spasticity or strength) does not directly translate into functional (dis)abilities or more "higher-level" issues, such as quality of life. Thus, some of the usual assumptions about health-related outcome measurement are not fully applicable in CP. Understanding issues such as change or the importance of individual preferences and goals in CP becomes even more salient when CP is viewed as a disability.

CURRENT OUTCOME ASSESSMENT IN CP

In the last 10 years, perspectives on outcome assessment in cerebral palsy have been influenced and shaped by the World Health Organization's International Classification of Functioning, Disability, and Health (ICF)[3] as a guiding principle. This seminal work describes and codifies a unifying means of understanding health status. The 2001 version for adults was followed in 2007 by an ICF for children and youth.[4] The ICF is a framework that captures the breadth of issues created by CP and the many arenas of impact. In brief, the ICF considers that each person's function, disability, and health are interdependent and are modified by environmental and personal factors. Thus, the ICF provides descriptions in 3 major domains of body function, body structure, and activities and participation (execution of tasks and activities and involvement in a life situation). These domains are further classified with contextual factors, either personal or environmental. ICF domains have been used to understand and describe the many impacts of CP for individuals and allow for categorization of various CP outcome measures by the domain that is being assessed.

Use of the ICF in CP outcome measurement might best be understood with an example. Consider the use of botulinum toxin in a child with diparetic CP and an abnormal gait. A range of concepts across the ICF spectrum might be altered by the use of botulinum toxin, and each of these concepts could be assessed using different outcome measures or assessment tools. In the domain of body structure, botulinum toxin might have no effects, but it might change muscle structure or create cortical reorganization that could be detected with muscle biopsy or functional magnetic resonance imaging (fMRI). In the domain of body function, changes in spasticity and strength could be measured with the Tardieu or Ashworth scales and dynamometry. Activity and participation is a single domain but may best be considered in 2 parts. Activity for a child with spastic diparesis might be altered with botulinum toxin by changing gross motor skills or gait pattern, which could be assessed with the Gross Motor Function Measure[5] or an observational gait scale. Participation realms would include playing on a sports team or attending more social events, which might be measured with the Children's Assessment of Participation and Enjoyment.[6] Environmental contextual factors, unlikely to be changed by botulinum toxin treatment, would include things such as accessible facilities and transportation to medical appointments. This example demonstrates the use of the ICF in capturing the range of issues for children with CP.

The attention to these concepts has resulted in greater understanding of the relationships among the domains of the ICF in CP. Most notably, recent work has demonstrated that there are no fixed relationships among the domains of the ICF. Although improvement at the level of body function and activity may take place (eg, decreased spasticity and better gross motor function), this does not necessarily mean improved participation or family satisfaction.[7] Furthermore, severity of impairment or disability is not directly correlated with quality of life.[8] These findings have been best interpreted in the light of the ICF.

Choosing the most appropriate outcome measures or assessment tools in clinical research or the clinical care of CP is challenging. With a vast array of areas of interest, many tools have been developed and are being used. Many outcome measures in use are fairly specific for 1 domain of the ICF, whereas others may span 2 or more domains. Some measures have been carefully designed, validated, and found to be reliable, whereas others were developed casually and have not been evaluated for their performance. Clinicians and researchers must think critically about the available tests, studies, questionnaires, evaluations, interviews, and technologies, and they must consider the patient or subject, the situation, and the question at hand before making selections.

When considering outcome measures, it is necessary to evaluate the psychometric performance of each measure. The best measure is one that addresses the domain of concern, is validated and reliable, can be applied readily, and is responsive to change. For many measures, some of these criteria are not yet fulfilled. Validity and reliability are key concepts in outcome measurement that demonstrate that the measure truly assesses the concepts of interest and that the assessments are accurate and repeatable. Many measures in use for children with CP have been evaluated for validity and reliability in at least a preliminary fashion. Even so, caution must be paid to using each instrument in the manner it was intended, which means administering each measure precisely as the developers instruct, including avoiding the use of tool subscales if the subscales have not been demonstrated to stand alone, using the measure in intended populations, and administering the measure as recommended. Some measures are best described as classifications. For example, the Gross Motor Function Classification System (GMFCS) delineates 5 strata of motor functioning in children and youth with CP.[9] It is convenient and widely used to describe severity of impairment in CP, but it has not been demonstrated to be useful to detect changes with time or after interventions, and it was not designed for this purpose. The ability to pick up differences with time is called responsiveness or sensitivity to change. This concept is not well studied for most CP outcome measures. Some measures require special equipment, trained assessors, or lengthy periods of administration; these measures may be less attractive to use because of the costs or inconveniences associated with them.

An additional concern for choosing outcome measures in CP research is the need for appropriate study design. The desire for greater information about clinical prognosis, natural history, and effects of intervention is great, and many researchers strive to provide answers. Unfortunately, if studies are not designed well, much effort and many resources may be expended without yielding useful evidence to advance knowledge. In CP research, many studies lack basic design elements, such as defining a primary outcome measure (the main thing that the study intends to evaluate for change) or power calculations (to assure that the study has the right number of subjects to answer the research question). Many studies do not create high-level evidence because they do not use high-quality design features, including randomization, blinding, allocation concealment, prospective recruitment, and adequate follow-up periods. Thus, without care in study design, the selection of the perfect outcome measure does not assure that a study is of value.

EXAMPLES OF COMMON OUTCOME MEASURES USED IN CP CLINICAL CARE AND RESEARCH

Dozens of measures are used in the care and research of childhood CP. The items discussed later are some of the more common outcome measures and are provided as examples. The list is in no way exhaustive, nor should it be interpreted as a "best available" list. A primary tenet of this article is the concept that outcome measurement in CP is complex, and decisions about which assessments should be used must be informed by the patient population and the goals of the evaluation. Measures are reviewed based on the primary ICF domain that they address. Measures of body structure and function selected address the primary condition of CP and not the secondary or associated conditions.

Body structure is not commonly evaluated in CP clinical trials. Although most children will have brain imaging to support their diagnoses of CP, subsequent evaluations are infrequent. In some settings, particularly for research, fMRI is used. fMRI explores brain activity during functional tasks. Little is known about how fMRI findings relate to other outcomes or how they could be applied clinically. Limited data have demonstrated reliability of fMRI findings in some populations.[10,11] Because fMRI is expensive and can be performed only in specialty centers, this technology is not widely used at present.

Body function is a frequent arena for CP outcome measures. Spasticity treatments are common in CP care and various means of evaluation include the Ashworth and Tardieu scales. Scores using these scales are determined by physically moving joints and describing the ease and range of movement. The Ashworth and Modified Ashworth Scales have limited reliability, and their validity is largely not proved (in part because spasticity has long been challenging to quantify).[12] The Tardieu scale may be somewhat less unreliable.[13] Despite the obvious shortcomings of these spasticity measures, they are almost universally used in clinical and research settings for CP, due to lack of better-performing assessments of spasticity that are easy to use. Strength is often measured using dynamometry. Various dynamometers and techniques are available to directly measure force generation, and some are easier to use or are more reliable than others. In general, ratings for most muscle groups are reliable.[14] Strength measurement is used variably in therapy settings and for some research. Range of motion may be assessed with goniometry, using a handheld device held alongside a child's limb to measure angles. Goniometry varies in reliability in research settings for children with CP,[15,16] although it continues to be used in clinical settings.

Activity measures are less frequently used in clinical settings, probably because of the time and training required for administration. The Gross Motor Function Measure is a therapist-administered battery of physical tasks that has established reliability and validity.[17] It takes an hour to complete but provides interval data quantifying a child's status that can be compared with motor development curves for CP.[18] The Pediatric Evaluation of Disability Inventory is a structured interview that generates scores in arenas of self-care, mobility, and social functioning,[19] with evidence of reliability, validity, and responsiveness.

The Canadian Occupational Performance Measure may be assigned to the activity or participation domains. It assesses an individual's perspective on his or her tasks of daily life and leisure as well as the individual's satisfaction with his or her performance.[20] This measure is fairly unique because it creates individualized priorities rather than evaluating the same tasks or actions for each participant. Reliability, validity, and responsiveness are established.

Most participation measures in use for children have adequate reliability and validity,[21] with less demonstrated responsiveness. The Children's Assessment of Participation and Enjoyment examines what activities and interests a child is pursuing and the child's enjoyment of the things she does.[6] This survey catalogs information about 55 activities, including what, where, when, and how often to describe participation.

General health or health status measures include several questionnaires. Some are generic measures that are broadly applied to pediatric populations, which include the Pediatric Quality of Life Inventory,[22] a questionnaire with physical and psychosocial subscales that may be completed by the child or a parent proxy. Another generic measure is the Kidscreen, which addresses health-related quality of life with a questionnaire, again available for children or parents.[23] Among the disease-specific health status measures are the Cerebral Palsy Quality of Life Questionnaire for Children (CP-QOL)[24] and the Caregiver Priorities and Child Health Index of Life with Disabilities (CPCHILD).[25] The CP-QOL is a questionnaire, for parent or child to complete, directed at quality of life in general rather than the more specific concept of health-related quality of life. The CPCHILD measures health status and burden-of-care for children with severe impairments and is completed by the parent. All of these questionnaires have been evaluated for validity and reliability.

Lastly, classification measures have become common mechanisms for describing children with CP in the last several years. In lieu of anatomic descriptions of CP, such as spastic diplegia or total body involvement, researchers and clinicians have adopted function-based classifications. The most common schema is the GMFCS.[9] The GMFCS is reliable, stable, and easy to use, such that parents can accurately classify children with CP into the 5 strata of functioning.[26] The highest functioning stratum, I, includes children who walk without restrictions, but have limitations in advanced motor skills. The lowest stratum is V and includes children who have severely limited self-mobility, even with assistive technology.[9] Similar classification systems have been developed for manual abilities[27] and communication.[28]

UNDERSTANDING CHANGE IN CEREBRAL PALSY

Evaluating change is the primary reason to measure outcomes. Clinicians, researchers, and especially children and parents want to know if things are different. In CP, understanding change is a complex endeavor. Interventions for CP are not curative, at least with current medical science. This means that one must look for changes in the symptoms or impacts of CP, but one does not expect dramatic resolution of CP or its associated disability. Assessing changes in CP involves evaluating more subtle changes than in some other diagnoses, such as having a lower blood pressure after taking medication. As was reviewed earlier, most individuals with CP have multiple domains of concern that range across the ICF.

Even within any given domain, assessing change requires careful study. Children with CP are truly moving targets. Their function and well-being are expected to change as they grow, develop, and mature. Some of these changes are the result of typical development and may mirror typically developing children; other changes are a direct consequence of the impairments of CP. These changes are often described as the natural history of CP. As children with CP are expected to change, any change that is established over time may simply be the result of natural maturation or development. The pace and degree of change are generally not sufficiently understood to make highly reliable predictions. Without this ability to prognosticate accurately, clinicians and researchers cannot establish if changes that follow a treatment for CP are the result of the treatment or are just "natural history." When working with populations of children with CP, studies that use randomized designs control for this issue, but otherwise it is almost impossible to differentiate the effects of interventions from the effects of development in CP.

Another tension in defining change in CP is the issue of significance. Research may be conducted to evaluate an intervention, and the results may indicate a statistical effect. This statistical effect would reflect a mathematical likelihood that change occurred with the intervention in terms of the outcome measurements. This mathematical happenstance, however, may or may not reflect a sufficient clinical change to justify the intervention. This concern is not frequent in CP research because of small sample sizes in most studies, but it remains salient. Consider a study that demonstrated a statistically significant improvement in knee-knee distance after botulinum toxin injection to the hip adductors.[29] The increase in knee separation was statistically analyzed and had changed from before to after, with an average increase of 10 cm. Some people would argue that increasing separation between knees by such a distance is not enough to make positioning, dressing, or diaper changes truly better. This could be an example of a finding that is statistically significant but not clinically significant.

When measuring change, some sort of ruler must be used. In CP research, many different outcome measures are used in this capacity. Most instruments have been evaluated to confirm that they truly measure what they are intended to measure and have established validity. Many of them, however, have not been evaluated for responsiveness. In an ideal setting, an outcome measure would be used in a population of subjects who are expected to show change to varying degrees. Additional means of evaluating change, maybe even a "gold standard," would be used concurrently with the outcome measure, and the data from each type of assessment would be compared. If the outcome measure scores changed in similar ways and with similar scope to the other assessments, then the outcome measure could be declared sensitive to change. Most measures used in CP have not been evaluated in this fashion. Thus, the numbers of outcome measures that have clearly demonstrated adequate responsiveness are low.

Tied to the idea of responsiveness is the concept of minimal clinically important differences (MCIDs). These differences are the amount a score on a measure needs to increase or decrease to reflect a change in status that is appreciable at a clinical level.[30] The best way to define these differences is to follow individuals with repeated evaluations with the measure that is being studied and with some other means to establish if the individual has changed in a meaningful manner. Outcome measure scores from the subjects who experience minimal clinical changes are then used to calculate the MCID. When this calculation has been made and a meaningful change score is defined, it is easier to better design studies in terms of selecting sample sizes, because the power calculations are straightforward. Secondly, clinical care is better informed when change scores can be compared with established MCIDs. See the article by Oeffinger and colleagues in this issue for studies to date that have aimed to establish MCIDs using instruments in wide use for CP.

SUMMARY

Outcome measurement may be the greatest hurdle in the research and clinical management of CP. Fortunately, greater appreciation now exists for the necessity of good outcome measures. With attention to the vast number of impacts of CP, the variability of CP manifestations, and the needs for valid, reliable, and responsive means of measuring the status of children with CP, more outcome measures are being investigated for their utility. The wise application of available outcome measures in optimized settings and thoughtful studies will lead to greater understanding of children with CP and the best management of their disabilities.

REFERENCES

1. Arnaud C, White-Koning M, Michelsen SI, et al. Parent-reported quality of life of children with cerebral palsy in Europe. Pediatrics 2008;121:54–64.
2. Raina P, O'Donnell M, Rosenbaum P, et al. The health and well-being of care-givers of children with cerebral palsy. Pediatrics 2005;115:e626–36.
3. World Health Organization. The international classification of functioning, disability and health (ICF). Geneva (Switzerland): World Health Organization; 2001.
4. World Health Organization. International classification of functioning, disability and health—children & youth version (ICF-CY). Geneva (Switzerland): World Health Organization; 2007.
5. Russell DJ, Rosenbaum PL, Avery LM, et al. Gross Motor Function Measure (GMFM-66 and GMFM-88) user's manual. In: Clinics in developmental medicine, vol. 15. London: MacKeith Press; 2002.
6. King GA, Law M, King S, et al. Measuring children's participation in recreation and leisure activities: construct validation of the CAPE and PAC. Child Care Health Dev 2007;33:28–39.
7. Bjornson K, Hays R, Graubert C, et al. Botulinum toxin for spasticity in children with cerebral palsy: a comprehensive evaluation. Pediatrics 2007;120:49–58.
8. Dickinson HO, Parkinson KN, Ravens-Sieberer U, et al. Self-reported quality of life of 8–12-year-old children with cerebral palsy: a cross-sectional European study. Lancet 2007;369:2171–8.
9. Palisano R, Rosenbaum P, Walter S, et al. Development and reliability of a system to classify gross motor function in children with cerebral palsy. Dev Med Child Neurol 1997;39:214–23.
10. Caceres A, Hall DL, Zelaya FO, et al. Measuring fMRI reliability with the intra-class correlation coefficient. Neuroimage 2008;45:758–68.
11. Kimberley TJ, Khandekar G, Borich M. fMRI reliability in subjects with stroke. Exp Brain Res 2008;186:183–90.
12. Clopton N, Dutton J, Featherston T, et al. Interrater and intrarater reliability of the modified Ashworth scale in children with hypertonia. Pediatr Phys Ther 2005;17: 268–74.
13. Haugh AB, Pandyan AD, Johnson GR. A systematic review of the Tardieu Scale for the measurement of spasticity. Disabil Rehabil 2006;28:899–907.
14. Crompton J, Galea MP, Phillips B. Hand-held dynamometry for muscle strength measurement in children with cerebral palsy. Dev Med Child Neurol 2007;49: 106–11.
15. Glanzman AM, Swenson AE, Kim H. Intrarater range of motion reliability in cere-bral palsy: a comparison of assessment methods. Pediatr Phys Ther 2008;20: 369–72.
16. Ten Berge SR, Halbertsma JP, Maathuis PG, et al. Reliability of popliteal angle measurement: a study in cerebral palsy patients and healthy controls. J Pediatr Orthop 2007;27:648–52.

17. Russell DJ, Avery LM, Rosenbaum PL, et al. Improved scaling of the gross motor function measure for children with cerebral palsy: evidence of reliability and validity. Phys Ther 2000;80:873–85.
18. Rosenbaum PL, Walter SD, Hanna SE, et al. Prognosis for gross motor function in cerebral palsy: creation of motor development curves. JAMA 2002;288:1357–63.
19. Haley S, Coster W, Ludlow L. Pediatric evaluation of disability inventory (PEDI), version 1: development, standardization and administration manual. Boston (MA): New England Medical Center, PEDI Research Group; 1992.
20. Law M, Baptiste S, McColl M, et al. The Canadian occupational performance measure: an outcome measure for occupational therapy. Can J Occup Ther 1990;57:82–7.
21. Sakzewski L, Boyd R, Ziviani J. Clinimetric properties of participation measures for 5- to 13-year-old children with cerebral palsy: a systematic review. Dev Med Child Neurol 2007;49:232–40.
22. Varni JW, Seid M, Kurtin PS. PedsQL 4.0: reliability and validity of the pediatric quality of life inventory version 4.0 generic core scales in healthy and patient populations. Med Care 2001;39:800–12.
23. Robitail S, Simeoni MC, Erhart M, et al. Validation of the European proxy KIDSCREEN-52 pilot test health-related quality of life questionnaire: first results. J Adolesc Health 2006;39:596 e1–10.
24. Waters E, Davis E, Reddihough D, et al. A new condition specific quality of life scale for children with cerebral palsy. PRO Newsletter 2005;35:10–2.
25. Narayanan UG, Fehlings D, Weir S, et al. Initial development and validation of the caregiver priorities and child health index of life with disabilities (CPCHILD). Dev Med Child Neurol 2006;48:804–12.
26. Palisano R, Cameron D, Rosenbaum P, et al. Stability of the gross motor function classification system. Dev Med Child Neurol 2004;99(Suppl 46):4 [abstract].
27. Eliasson AC, Krumlinde-Sundholm L, Rosblad B, et al. The Manual Ability Classification System (MACS) for children with cerebral palsy: scale development and evidence of validity and reliability. Dev Med Child Neurol 2006;48:549–54.
28. Hidecker MJC, Paneth N, Rosenbaum P, et al. Developing a classification tool of functional communication in individuals with cerebral palsy. Dev Med Child Neurol 2008;50:43.
29. Mall V, Heinen F, Siebel A, et al. Treatment of adductor spasticity with BTX-A in children with CP: a randomized, double-blind, placebo-controlled study. Dev Med Child Neurol 2006;48:10–3.
30. Beaton DE, Bombardier C, Katz JN, et al. Looking for important change/differences in studies of responsiveness. OMERACT MCID Working group. Outcome measures in rheumatology minimal clinically important difference. J Rheumatol 2001;28:400–5.

Parent–Professional Partnership

Cynthia Frisina Gray, MA, MBA[a], Melissa Siebert, JD, MBA[a],
Mindy Aisen, MD, CEO[b], Deborah Gaebler-Spira, MD[c,d],*

KEYWORDS

- Cerebral palsy • Parents • Advocacy
- Research • Communication

Rehabilitation management of children with cerebral palsy (CP) brings together parents and doctors. The primary goal of the contact is to improve the individual child's potential and to improve the child's functional outcomes. Frequently, parents are interested in not just their own child, but the population of children with CP. Physicians can provide information for both purposes. Successful parent–professional relationships are rewarding and powerful. Combining the passion of the parent and the expertise of the physician can enhance collaboration for advocacy efforts that improve outcomes for children with CP.

This article (1) reviews essential aspects of communication, (2) discusses the importance of parent networks, (3) encourages collaboration of physicians and parents as a force for advocacy, and (4) provides information on organizations that can help physicians develop the skills to be effective advocates.

COMMUNICATION

The medical encounter consists of 2 experts: the parent and the physician. The parent knows more than anyone about the child and the family; the physician brings medical expertise and experience. The medical visit is based on communication between these 2 experts. Of all the skills of a physician, listening is the key to understanding the experience of the child and the parent.

---

[a] "Reaching For The Stars. A Foundation of Hope for Children with Cerebral Palsy" (RFTS, Inc.), 3000 Old Alabama Road, Suite 119-300, Alpharetta, GA 30022, USA
[b] Georgetown University of Medicine, 1025 Connecticut NW, Washington, DC, USA
[c] Department of Pediatrics, Northwestern University, Chicago, IL, USA
[d] Department of Physical Medicine and Rehabilitation, Northwestern University, Chicago, IL, USA
* Corresponding author. Pediatric Rehabilitation Program, Department of Physical Medicine and Rehabilitation, Rehabilitation Institute of Chicago, 345 East Superior, Suite 1160, Chicago, IL 60611.
E-mail addresses: dgaebler@ric.org (D. Gaebler-Spira); www.reachingforthestars.org (RFTS, Inc.).

Phys Med Rehabil Clin N Am 20 (2009) 577–585
doi:10.1016/j.pmr.2009.04.001
1047-9651/09/$ – see front matter © 2009 Elsevier Inc. All rights reserved.

pmr.theclinics.com

Talk forms the basis of the encounter; however, the importance of talking is often underestimated. Most medical historians agree that talking has shifted away from the center of the encounter. Shorter[1] identified the post–World War II era (coinciding with the development of antibiotics) as the time that the disease rather than the patient's experience became the focus of the encounter. The practice of linear interviewing, with yes/no questions as the format of conversation, curtails the opportunity for support and discussion of social aspects of the condition. This is reflected in a study focusing on the first 90 seconds of the patient encounter, in which the patient's response to the first question was completed only 23% of the time, and physicians interrupted the response after an average of 15 seconds.[2]

A small observational study compared internal medicine physicians using electronic medical records with those using paper records.[3] Although the study did not identify statistically significant differences, it suggested that physicians using electronic medical records were less likely than other physicians to attend to psychosocial issues and the patient's experience of an illness.

In the conversation between the physician and the parent of a child with CP, providing appropriate care often depends on a shared perception of the problem that needs attention. A particular constraint of the electronic medical record may be a decreased opportunity to assess a parent's perception of the evolving needs of a child with a chronic neurologic disorder such as CP.

Rehabilitation management takes into account the model of outcome of the International Classification of Functioning, Disability and Health (ICF) (**Fig. 1**).[4] The continuum of body structures and function, activities, and participation creates opportunities to look beyond health status and assist with integration into the community. The patient encounter in rehabilitation includes all dimensions of the ICF model. The model encompasses the personal and external factors that affect the more traditional biomedical model of body structure/body functions, activities, and participation categories. Personal factors that affect outcome include access to information and

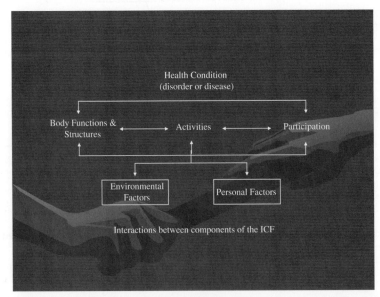

Fig. 1. World Health Organization International Classification of Function, Disability and Health. (*Data from* World Health Organization. International classification of functioning, disability and health. Available at: http://www.who.int/classifications/icf/en/. Accessed February 14, 2009.)

networking support for parents and children. External factors include the societal barriers that may impede participation, such as health care disparity, educational barriers, and lack of adequate funding for research in CP at the national level. Communication that is free flowing is necessary to gather information that touches on all aspects of the ICF model. Nonlinear communication favors obtaining the psychosocial component that brings the personal and environmental barriers to the fore. When the patient and the professional have equal control of the communication, a mutual relationship exists. This mutual relationship is considered ideal.[5] This *system of care* and communication approach to CP is changing the relationship of parents to members of their child's medical team at every level. The collaboration of families and medical professionals is now recognized as a best practice for many other disorders, including autism, muscular dystrophy, and cystic fibrosis. These collaborative partnerships have resulted in measurable and direct positive benefits for families, children, and medical providers.

These issues may be considered in light of a set of positive principles that inform the style of communication in the medical encounter. Communication should serve the patient's need to tell the story and the doctor's need to hear it; highlight the knowledge and insight of the patient about illness and well-being; reflect the doctor's understanding of the connection between mental and physical health; proceed in a way that gives the doctor a chance to use experience and expertise to assist the child and the family; take into account the emotional impact of the encounter; be an opportunity to negotiate what is desired by both patient and physician; overcome stereotyped roles; and strengthen the relationship of patient and physician.[5] When positive communication is encouraged, physicians elicit personal factors that affect rehabilitation. By understanding the parent's knowledge-base, the physician can suggest appropriate educational and parental support.

IMPORTANCE OF PARENT'S NETWORKS

Parents raising a child with CP often experience anxiety, frustration, and isolation. It can be overwhelming to navigate the medical and educational systems, and sometimes the legal system, along with completing the tasks of daily life. Sharing experiences with others in similar circumstances is a source of relief and lessens the sense of isolation. There is an automatic understanding of the visceral and practical issues that accompanies being a caregiver of a child with CP. It is because of this "automatic understanding" that parents of children with CP prefer to receive emotional support from other parents who have had or who are having the same or similar experiences.

Medical and rehabilitation services for children with CP are generally time limited, whereas the family and the community are constants in a child's life. Drawing effectively on parent and community resources enhances the likelihood that medical and therapeutic treatments combined with family support will promote better outcomes. Professionals and families working together can create home- and community-based alternatives that supplement formal services and provide structure, nurturing, and support. As budgets shrink and needs grow, parent advocacy and involvement can help decrease the workload of the professional by expanding the treatment options.

WHO BENEFITS?

A quantitative study of parent-to-parent support groups showed that parents who participated in these groups had a greater increase in measures of cognitive adaptation and coping than parents in a control group. In addition, 89% of parents reported that the program was helpful.[6] Families report that after becoming involved with organizations such as *Reaching For The Stars. A Foundation of Hope for Children with Cerebral Palsy* (www.reachingforthestars.org), Pathways, Easter Seals, and United Cerebral Palsy, they receive services earlier, identify more community resources, and understand parenting issues more clearly. The Beach Center on Disability at the University of Kansas (www.beachcenter.org), a respected research institution, Family Support America (FamilySupportAmerica.org), and the National Federation of Families for Children's Mental Health (ffcmh.org) all acknowledge the benefits of family involvement and advocacy (**Box 1**).

Parents as Advocates

Parent advocacy is a respected and effective strategy to provide support and education to families of children with CP. It is only one component in a continuum of family involvement, but it has gained wide use in other disorders affecting children.

Advocacy is defined as "speaking for another person or cause." Because of the complex issues surrounding parenting children with CP, many families need support in acting as advocates for themselves and their children.

Parent advocates can also push for research funding, which will lead to information about etiology, prevention, and effective treatment, improving the ability of physicians to provide effective and efficient care for patients and families. Advocacy is an integral part of the mission for parent groups like *Reaching For The Stars. A Foundation of Hope for Children with Cerebral Palsy* (reachingforthestars.org), the only national, nonprofit pediatric cerebral palsy foundation led by parents in the U.S. The foundation's mission is centered on the belief that advocacy, parent education and leading-edge pediatric research can lead to new treatments of CP and deliver measurable improvements in the lives of impacted children and their families. RFTS, Inc. conducts parent education conferences around the country in conjunction with major medical institutions, in addition to advocacy and supporting clinical trial research.

This partnership is the thread that links successful practices, new treatments, and standards of care for children with CP. Parents are now acting as advocates for change; mentors to other families; and active participants in clinical, public service, and legislative programs and policies.

Since CP is the most common cause of motor disability in childhood, parents are concerned about prevention, treatment, socio-educational issues, and long-term

Box 1
Parents as advocates

Benefits	
For Families	**For Medical Professionals**
Increases knowledge of their child's disorder	Allows more efficiency in care of child
Provides opportunities to network with other families	Saves money by extending resources
Increases confidence in parenting skills	Improves quality of service
Increases knowledge and skills	Develops additional advocates and a shared burden of care
Creates a sense of belonging	Decreases workload
Increases sense of personal power	Contributes to the stability of the community

outcomes for their children. A newly published multisite study of CP in the United States[7] reported a prevalence of 3.6 for every 1000 8-year-old children (approximately 1 in 278 children). This is considerably more than the previous estimated prevalence of 1 in 666 children. Recent scientific advances in the understanding of brain development and plasticity offer hope for increasing understanding of this disorder and stimulating the development of novel strategies to optimize functioning—but this will not happen without funding to attract and support the scientists needed to provide these breakthroughs.

This new report also serves as another reminder to parents of how medicine in the United States, with a focus on cutting-edge treatments, can fail hundreds of thousands of children affected by a common yet complex disorder. Medical researchers are still unsure about the causes of CP. However, 2 of the top risk factors—premature births and multiple births—have increased in the United States despite advances in prenatal testing, improved obstetric care, and newborn intensive care technologies.

COLLABORATION: PARENTS AND PROFESSIONALS

Parents of children with CP have joined forces with medical professionals and have begun to take organized steps toward affecting national policy and funding initiatives. Parent advocates from *Reaching For The Stars. A Foundation of Hope for Children with Cerebral Palsy* (www.reachingforthestars.org), in conjunction with organizations such as the Cerebral Palsy International Research Foundation, the American Academy for Cerebral Palsy and Developmental Medicine, and the Child Neurology Society, have been instrumental in urging Congress to fund national CP surveillance and epidemiologic research. Through these collaborative efforts, support of key senators was established, and a congressional report was recently issued to look at funding needs for CP research. There is also a Senate bill (with bipartisan sponsorship) identifying March 25 as National Cerebral Palsy Awareness Day.

COLLABORATIVE RESEARCH—IMPORTANT PARTNERSHIP

Another key area of parent–medical professional collaboration is fostering the expansion of pediatric CP research, both locally and nationally. These collaborations can be in the form of direct funding, advocacy at a state and national level for funding (Centers for Disease Control and Prevention [CDC], National Institutes of Health [NIH], National Science Foundation [NSF]), and privately funded projects.

National funding for CP by the federal government has been minimal in comparison to funding for research for other prevalent disorders of childhood. In 2005, the NIH provided $60,000,000 for childhood leukemia (affecting 1 in 29,000) and $23,000,000 for CP (affecting 1 in 278). In the same year, the CDC provided $5,104,000 in federal funds for national spina bifida surveillance and $0 in federal funds for national surveillance for CP. The minimal level of federal funding (NIH) for CP research becomes readily apparent when compared with federal funding for other childhood conditions in terms of annual funding per new case. NIH funding for CP was estimated to be $28 million in fiscal year (FY) 2008. Estimates of CP prevalence in the western world range from 2 to 4.4 cases per 1000 live births.[8-12] As there were more than 4 million live births in the United States in 2005,[13] a reasonable estimate of the number of new cases of CP per year is 12,000. This results in approximately $2300 federal research dollars being spent annually for every new case of CP. In FY 2008, the NIH expended an estimated $90 million on cystic fibrosis research, $241 million on pediatric AIDS research, and $22 million on Duchenne/Becker muscular dystrophy research.[14] In the United States there are an estimated 0.3 new cases of cystic fibrosis per 1000 live births annually;[15] there were 135 new cases of pediatric AIDS reported to the CDC in 2006;[16] and the annual incidence of Duchenne muscular dystrophy has been estimated to be approximately 1 in 5618 male live births in the United Kingdom, whereas the incidence of Becker muscular dystrophy has been reported to be about one-third of that.[17] In contrast to funding for CP, it is estimated that annual federal funding per new case of cystic fibrosis, pediatric AIDS, and Duchenne/Becker muscular dystrophy is $41,000, $1.8 million, and $44,000, respectively.

The connection between private funding and CP research warrants more attention, particularly given the positive impact that private funding has had in advancements in the treatment of other, serious childhood conditions such as cystic fibrosis. Parental and foundation support has produced a strong national registry and funded research that has produced verifiable improvements in treatments and outcomes.

The history of private funding is clarified by United Cerebral Palsy (UCP) and Cerebral Palsy International Research Foundation. In 1955, UCP—an organization founded by parents of children with CP to help provide access to health care for those who could otherwise not afford it—created the UCP Research and Education Foundation. The mission of the foundation is to support research relevant to prevention, cure, and effective treatment of CP and its complications. In 2008, the UCP Research and Education Foundation became the Cerebral Palsy International Research Foundation (CPIRF). CPIRF funds original research worldwide on a merit-based system. In addition to bench research into causes and prevention of CP, emphasis is also being placed on new technologies for improving quality of life and developing direct treatment of the brain disorder (such as robotic and virtual reality techniques for promoting appropriate nervous system reorganization—capitalizing on the innate plasticity of the human nervous system), socioeconomic studies, and clinical trials. CPIRF provides information via the Internet and supports workshops for people with CP and their families, clinicians, and researchers to promote dialog and increase meaningful research.

CPIRF funds several workshops per year and supports 15 to 25 research projects each year (providing $50,000 per project for each of 2 years). CPIRF also grants 1 to 3 Hausman Awards per year for career development; the award is named after Ethel Hausman, one of the founders of the organization, and is given to fund junior investigators with clinical training in a mentored program.

The affiliates of UCP are local facilities that provide clinical, educational, and social services for children with disabilities, including CP; however, the majority of their clients do not have CP. Services provided differ from state to state.

Another instance of the impact of private funding is the development of the Cerebral Palsy Registry in the Chicago area (CPregistry.org). The purpose of the registry is to create a database of children with CP and to collect data on gestation, birth, genetic factors, medical and surgical history, motor function, services received, activities and participation, quality of life, and willingness to participate in research studies. The Cerebral Palsy Registry is a joint project involving the Rehabilitation Institute of Chicago, Northwestern University Feinberg School of Medicine's Department of Physical Therapy and Human Movement Sciences, the University of Chicago, La Rabida Children's Hospital, and Children's Memorial Hospital. Potential uses of data generated by such a registry are (1) creation of a database of available research study participants to support large research studies and gain federal funding; (2) increasing longitudinal data regarding the well-being, function, burden of care, and social participation of children growing into adulthood with CP; and (3) improving medical surveillance for better focus on treatment and research.

Another important example of parent–professional partnership to advance care of children with CP is the use of parent networks to recruit for clinical trials. The parent advocates of *Reaching For The Stars. A Foundation of Hope for Children with Cerebral Palsy* (reachingforthestars.org) are collaborating with investigators to encourage family participation in studies such as the use of baclofen in pediatric CP (the Baclofen Efficacy and Safety Trial: Pediatric Pharmacokinetic and Pharmacodynamic Study of Oral Baclofen for the Treatment of Spasticity Associated with Cerebral Palsy); they are also supporting studies on improvement of motor functioning in children with CP and a large-scale study examining the effectiveness of care received by children with CP. Many investigators leading these research efforts are making it a practice to collaborate with parents.

NEW FORMATS FOR ADVOCACY

Other key parent–medical partnership initiatives include developing and promoting new discoveries and clinical research programs to advance the pharmacologic, surgical, and therapeutic treatment of CP. For example, an initiative planned by the New York chapter of United Cerebral Palsy is the launching of www.mychildwithoutlimits.org, a comprehensive resource for information and social networking for families and caregivers of children aged 0 to 5 years with CP and other developmental disabilities, and for the professionals who work with them.

Another important resource is the Pathways Awareness Foundation, a national nonprofit organization dedicated to raising awareness about the benefit of early detection of motor delays and early therapy for children to help all children reach their fullest potential. The Pathways Web site, which is designed in collaboration with both parents and professionals, contains valuable information about children's physical development and crucial infant milestones.

Recognition of the increasing importance of the Internet as a source of information for parents is shown by the publication of a recent article entitled "'Is My Child Developing Normally?': A Critical Review of Web-Based Resources for Parents" in *Developmental Medicine and Child Neurology*.[18] The authors rated 44 Web sites for such components as content, design, navigability, layout, and readability. Overall, the authors found that the information on child development presented on the Web sites was accurate but often incomplete or difficult to understand.

OPPORTUNITIES FOR INVOLVEMENT

The physician can become involved with educational and advocacy groups in addition to individual professional societies. Most physicians are members of professional societies and participate in continuing education as a part of maintenance of certification programs and to satisfy requirements for state licensing. Because caring for children and adults with CP involves collaboration among multiple specialists, societies that blend specialties and educational opportunities are necessary. There are a few opportunities to participate in continuing education meetings that involve multiple disciplines and present high-quality research. Organizations at the national level providing such opportunities include the American Academy of Physical Medicine and Rehabilitation, the American Academy of Pediatrics Council on Developmental Disabilities, the American Academy for Cerebral Palsy and Developmental Medicine, and the Association of Children's Prosthetic-Orthotic Clinics; and at the international level they include the European Academy of Childhood Disability and the International Society for Prosthetics and Orthotics.

SUMMARY

An increasingly important component in the parent–medical collaboration is the identification of networks of local and national support for families of children with CP.

Fortunately, parents and organizations focused on children with CP are seeing the necessity for collaboration to build community awareness, implement education programs, and spearhead pediatric CP advocacy on a nationwide basis.

Advocacy for research funding is needed in both private and public arenas. Private research foundations can support the funding of innovative pilot projects. Federal funding should be increased to a level consistent with support for other prevalent disorders of childhood.

Development of an evidence-based approach for the treatment of CP is essential for good treatment and for reimbursement. Parents can be provided with information that will help them use their time and resources in management efforts that are likely to yield positive results.

Research is needed to document effective treatments and to understand the range of problems in this complex disorder. Ideas that stimulate research often depend on the ability of the parent to talk with the physician and the willingness of the physician to be an active listener. The concerns of the parents are essential in identifying the needs of children with CP. A parent–professional partnership that extends from the individual medical encounter to the development of national organizations can lead to achieving the goal of both sides of the partnership: improved care for children with CP.

REFERENCES

1. Shorter E. Bedside manners: the troubled history of doctors and patients. New York: Simon and Schuster; 1985.
2. Beckman HB, Frankel RM. The effect of physician behavior on the collection of data. Ann Intern Med 1984;101(5):692–6.
3. Makoul G, Curry RH, Tang PC. The use of electronic medical records. J Am Med Inform Assoc 2001;8:610–5.
4. World Health Organization. International classification of functioning, disability and health. Available at: http://www.who.int/classifications/icf/en/. Accessed February 14, 2009.
5. Roter D, Hall JA. Doctors talking with patients/patients talking with doctors: improving communication in medical visits. 2nd edition. Westport (CT): Praeger; 2006. p. 26.
6. Singer G, Marquis JG, Powers LK, et al. A multi-site evaluation of parent to parent programs for parents of children with disabilities. J Early Interv 1999;22:217–29.
7. Yeargin-Allsopp M, Van Naarden Braun K, Doernberg NS, et al. Prevalence of cerebral palsy in 8-year-old children in three areas of the United States in 2002: a multisite collaboration. Pediatrics 2008;121(3):547–54.
8. Surveillance of Cerebral Palsy in Europe (SCPE) Prevalence and characteristics of children with cerebral palsy in Europe. Dev Med Child Neurol 2002;44:633–40.
9. Uldall P, Michelson SI, Topp M, et al. The Danish Cerebral Palsy Registry. A registry on a specific impairment. Dan Med Bull 2001;48(3):161–3.
10. Hirtz D, Thurman DJ, Gwinn-Hardy K, et al. How common are the "common" neurologic disorders? Neurology 2007;68(5):326–37.
11. Serdaroglu A, Cansu A, Ozkan S, et al. Prevalence of cerebral palsy in Turkish children between the ages of 2 and 16 years. Dev Med Child Neurol 2006; 48(6):413–6.
12. Odding E, Roebroeck ME, Stam HJ. The epidemiology of cerebral palsy: incidence, impairments and risk factors. Disabil Rehabil 2006;28(4):183–91.
13. Martin JA, Hamilton BE, Sutton PD, et al. Births-Final Data for 2005 [report]. Hyattsville, MD: National Center for Health Statistics 2007;56(6).

14. NIH. NIH research portfolio online reporting tool. Available at: http://report.nih. gov/rcdc/categories/PFSummaryTable.aspx. Accessed February 14, 2009.
15. National Heart Lung and Blood Institute. Available at: http://www.nhlbi.nih.gov/ health/dci/Diseases/cf/cf_risk.html. Accessed February 14, 2009.
16. Centers for Disease Control HIV/AIDS surveillance report 2006; Vol 18 [report]. In: US Dept of Health and Human Services. Atlanta, GA: Centers for Disease Control and Prevention 2008. Available at: http://www.cdc.gov/hiv/topics/surveillance/ resources/reports. Accessed April 10, 2009.
17. Bushby KM, Thambyayah M, Gardner-Medwin D. Prevalence and incidence of Becker muscular dystrophy. Lancet 1991;337(8748):1022–4.
18. Williams N, Mughal S, Blair M. 'Is my child developing normally?': a critical review of web-based resources for parents. Dev Med Child Neurol 2008;50(12):893–7.

Index

Note: Page numbers of article titles are in **boldface** type.

A

Activity, in osteoporosis treatment in cerebral palsy, 503–504
ADDM CP Network. See *Autism and Developmental Disability Monitoring (ADDM) CP Network.*
Advocacy, formats for, in parent-professional partnership, 583
Advocate(s), parents as, 580–581
Age, gestational, as risk factor for cerebral palsy, 436–439
Ambulation, in cerebral palsy, factors influencing, 471
Ambulatory children, with cerebral palsy
    clinical applications of outcome tools in, **549–565.** See also *Cerebral palsy, ambulatory children with, clinical applications of outcome tools in.*
    lower extremity management for, clinical and research trends in, **469–491.** See also *Cerebral palsy, ambulatory children with, lower extremity management for.*
American Community Survey, of US Census Bureau, 539
Arthrodesis(es), for motor disorders in cerebral palsy, 485–486
Assisted reproduction, as risk factor for cerebral palsy, 439–440
Autism and Developmental Disability Monitoring (ADDM) CP Network, 425

B

Birth weight, as risk factor for cerebral palsy, 436–439
Bisphosphonate(s), in osteoporosis treatment in cerebral palsy, 504
Bladder, neurogenic, in adult with cerebral palsy, management of, 514–515
Bone(s)
    absorption of, 495
    anatomy of, 494–495
    architecture of, 494–495
    composition of, 494–495
    embryology of, 494–495
    formation of, 495
    health of
        assessment of, 497–500
        in cerebral palsy, 500–502
    metabolism of, markers of, 495–496
    structure of, 494–495
Bone density
    assessment of
        DXA in, 497–499
        in cerebral palsy, challenges associated with, 500
        pQCT in, 499–500
        risks associated with, 500

Phys Med Rehabil Clin N Am 20 (2009) 587–594
doi:10.1016/S1047-9651(09)00045-X
1047-9651/09/$ – see front matter © 2009 Elsevier Inc. All rights reserved.

pmr.theclinics.com

Moving?

Make sure your subscription moves with you!

To notify us of your new address, find your **Clinics Account Number** (located on your mailing label above your name), and contact customer service at:

E-mail: elspcs@elsevier.com

800-654-2452 (subscribers in the U.S. & Canada)
314-453-7041 (subscribers outside of the U.S. & Canada)

Fax number: 314-523-5170

Elsevier Periodicals Customer Service
11830 Westline Industrial Drive
St. Louis, MO 63146

*To ensure uninterrupted delivery of your subscription, please notify us at least 4 weeks in advance of move.